Praise for Dr Atkinson

I regard Dr Mark Atkinson as the UK's leading visionary within the field of integrative medicine.

Professor Karol Sikora, Professor of Cancer Medicine

Praise for *True Happiness*

Dr Mark Atkinson is an acclaimed medical and integrated health practitioner – this gives his thesis gravitas – but most importantly his passion for health, well-being, joy and happiness are infectious. This book should be prescribed to all!

Janey Lee Grace, TV and radio presenter and author of
Imperfectly Natural Woman

This wonderful book combines wisdom, depth and readability. In it, Dr Mark Atkinson has mapped out a practical pathway to greater happiness, fulfilment and emotional skilfulness.

Dr Chris Johnstone, author of *Find Your Power – A Toolkit for Resilience and Positive Change*

Many people muddle through life in a partial coma, accepting a level of happiness and fulfillment that is only a fraction of their potential. With only a slight change in perspective, a new life awaits. If you aspire to live life fully, deeply, vitally, Dr Mark Atkinson's book is for you.

Larry Dossey, MD, author of *The Power of Premonitions* and *Healing Words* and executive editor of *Explore: The Journal of Science and Healing*

At last we have a truly comprehensive handbook on how to evolve physically, psychologically, and spiritually. This is a valuable toolbox to help us take care of ourselves. Dr Atkinson speaks not only as a teacher but as an encouraging companion on the path, so I felt somehow held and guided at the same time.

David Richo, PhD, author of *Daring to Trust: Opening Ourselves to Real Love and Intimacy*

True Happiness is a practical step-by-step guide to identifying and clearing the common blockages which stand in the way of real happiness. Full of sound psychology and wise advice, its eight pillars will guide you towards thinking and acting in ways that support your mental and physical health, and help you to create healthy and life-affirming relationships with others. Mark Atkinson reminds us that happiness does not come from outer success or circumstances. True happiness comes from within – and begins with self-love and acceptance of what is. This inspirational and heart-centred guide shows you how to get there.

Gill Edwards, clinical psychologist and author of *Conscious Medicine*

Congratulations, Dr Mark, on developing and sharing so effectively an approach to help us all achieve true happiness. Your astute mapping of the territory to lead us to happiness, your valuable self-assessment questions, and your effective solutions will help many, many people to a life of fulfilment and happiness. Wish I'd learnt this in my teens.

Dr Andrew Tresidder MBBS MRCGP, GP, author and educator

With remarkable depth and wisdom, Dr Atkinson shows us how to find complete fulfillment in life. In vivid detail, this book offers reliable practices that transform our negative emotions, attitudes and thinking that imprison us in a state of unease. Such a rare jewel for integrating our mind, body and spirit!

Jacquelyn Small, author of *The Sacred Purpose of Being Human, Transformers*, and *Awakening in Time*

Praise for Dr Atkinson's previous books
Holistic Health Secrets for Women

Holistic Health Secrets for Women is superb. It's loaded with practical and highly useful information that will help women of all ages look and feel their best.

Christiane Northrup, MD, author of *The Wisdom of Menopause* and *Women's Bodies, Women's Wisdom*

Whether you are looking for advice on a specific medical condition, or you simply want to improve your level of physical and emotional well being, this accessible and rousing book will inspire you to transform your health and your life.

Natural Products

An inspirational quick reference guide to steer you through the many conditions that may inflict the female of the species.

Yoga magazine

The Mind–Body Bible

The Mind–Body Bible is an excellent resource for those inspired individuals who seek empowerment and the knowledge to participate more fully in creating health and wellness. It is filled with information which is easy to understand and put to use in one's daily life. So read on and find your personalised pathway to health and well being.

Bernie Siegel, MD, author of *Love, Medicine & Miracles* and *Prescriptions for Living*

In *The Mind–Body Bible* Dr Atkinson has presented a new personalised model of integrated health, one that explores and provides comprehensive solutions to 14 of the most common physical, environmental, emotional and spiritual barriers to total health. His book will become a must-read for anyone who wants to transform their health and lead a more fulfilling life.

Kenneth R. Pelletier, PhD, MD(hc), author of *Best Alternative Medicine: What Works? What Does Not?*

TRUE HAPPINESS

Dr Mark Atkinson

Your complete guide
to emotional health

piatkus

PIATKUS

First published in Great Britain in 2011 by Piatkus
Copyright © Mark Atkinson 2011

The moral right of the author has been asserted.

A CIP catalogue record for this book
is available from the British Library.

ISBN 978-0-7499-2916-9

Typeset in Stone Serif by Phoenix Photosetting, Chatham, Kent
Printed and bound in Great Britain by MPG Books, Bodmin, Cornwall

Piatkus
An imprint of
Little, Brown Book Group
100 Victoria Embankment
London EC4Y 0DY

An Hachette UK Company
www.hachette.co.uk

www.piatkus.co.uk

Acknowledgements

I am grateful to the following individuals whose work, insights and guidance have inspired my own personal development and my professional work. They include: Michael Brown, Eckhart Tolle, Andrew Cohen, Arjuna Ardagh, Hal and Sidra Stone, Dennis Genpo Merzel, Deepak Chopra, David Simon, Gay Hendricks, Ken Wilber, Russ Harris, Pia Mellody, Janae and Barry Weinhold, Abraham Maslow, David Richo, Bill Plotkin, Byron Katie, Richard Miller, Stephen Bodian, Barbara Marx Hubbard and Duane Elgin.

And thank you to my agent, David, and the team at Piatkus, in particular Jillian Stewart, Gill Bailey and Anne Newman, for your support and expert guidance.

Contents

About the author

Dr Mark Atkinson is a medical doctor, holistic health and well-being expert and an internationally renowned authority on integrative medicine. He is also an inspiring teacher, workshop facilitator and founder of the Academy of Human Potential, one of the UK's leading personal development companies.

Dr Atkinson qualified as a medical doctor in 1997. On graduation, he received a MBBS (Bachelor of Medicine and Surgery) and a BSc HONS (Bachelor of Science in Clinical Pharmacology and Toxicology) from Imperial College School of Medicine in London (formerly St Mary's Hospital Medical School). As he worked with patients, Dr Atkinson became fascinated by the relationship between head, heart and body, and how they influence one another – for better or for worse. This inspired him to build on his conventional medical training and become involved in integrative medicine, which uses the most effective approaches and treatments from conventional and complementary medicine to bring about emotional and psychological – as well as physical – health. He continues to explore approaches that bring head, heart and body into balance and harmony, as it is this, he has discovered, that allows individuals to create the healthiest, happiest and most fulfilling life possible. This is the essence of his work today.

Dr Atkinson's unique approach has been endorsed by leading doctors, including Dr Andrew Weil, Dr Christiane Northrup, Professor Karol Sikora, Dr Bernie Siegel and Dr Larry Dossey. It has also been featured in the national press, including *The Daily Telegraph*, *The Mail on Sunday* and *The Sunday Times*. Dr Atkinson is also an award-winning writer and is the author of *The Mind–Body Bible* and *Holistic Health Secrets for Women*.

With this book, Dr Atkinson's aim is to help people realise their fullest potential by maximising their well-being and nurturing their emotional and spiritual intelligence. Indeed that is the mission of The Academy of Human Potential, which he founded in 2008. The Academy supports individuals in this through talks, workshops, coaching and consultation services, leadership development programmes and professional training courses. Through the Academy, he has trained a team of Human Potential coaches who have the skills and experience to support you through your own true happiness journey.

For more information on Dr Atkinson's approach, see www.drmarkatkinson.com. For more on discovering true happiness, including details of Dr Atkinson's course in true happiness, visit www.discovertruehappiness.com

Introduction

Are you fed up with the way you feel? Do you suffer from negative thoughts or over-thinking? Is guilt, anxiety, depression, anger, resentment or emotional pain preventing you from living the life you want to? Do you struggle to be yourself? Do you want to change your life and discover how to experience lasting true happiness?

If you answered 'Yes' to any of the above questions, you are in the right place. In the last ten years I have used my revolutionary approach to help hundreds of people transform their physical and emotional health and find what I call true happiness.

Before I explain what true happiness is let me first explain why, as a medical doctor, I am interested in happiness. The simple answer is this – happiness is one of the master keys to creating a healthy body and mind. And there is plenty of research to substantiate that. What's more, many of my patients have found that as they start to experience true happiness they feel more peaceful, joyful, creative and loving. Their relationships start to improve, they become more successful in what they do for a living and – maybe above all else – they start to feel a deeper sense of acceptance and connection to themselves and others. It turns out that if you want to awaken your highest potential for health, love and success, happiness is the key.

So how can I help you?

My passion is for helping individuals overcome any health challenges they may have and to support them in living the healthiest, happiest and most fulfilling life possible. If you are like most people, you've probably already tried various things – from meditation and self-help books to supplements, complementary therapies and medication – in an attempt to be happier and create a better life for yourself. You may well feel better as a result of these; however, because you are reading this book, I assume you are still looking for ways to feel happier and more fulfilled. So what can I offer that will work for you? What is unique about my approach?

- It works – it is based on my experience of helping hundreds of my patients discover a new level of health and happiness.

- Because I am an integrative medical doctor I take a big-picture overview of happiness and emotional health – one that covers body, mind, emotions, relationships and spirit (all of which need to be addressed in order to experience true happiness).

- It offers some of the most innovative self-help tools and techniques for personal growth and emotional healing. These are the tools and techniques that have worked for my patients.

- It's practical – questionnaires and easy-to-follow advice will help you overcome the most common physical barriers to emotional health and happiness. These include allergies/food intolerances, blood-sugar imbalances, nutrient deficiencies, hormone problems, dysbiosis (gut imbalance) and neurotransmitter imbalances. Despite being a factor in about 80 per cent of cases, most books on happiness and emotional health (particularly those written by psychologists and psychotherapists) fail to address these.

So why *true* happiness?

The desire for happiness is at the root of everything we do. Yet many of us look for happiness in the wrong place. We assume that success, status, money, achievements, people, places, possessions or power will bring us happiness. Of course they can and do influence for better or worse the way we feel, but this kind of 'normal' happiness comes and goes depending on what is happening in our lives and does not deliver lasting happiness and well-being. *True* happiness, in contrast, is less about what happens to us and more about living with greater awareness and acceptance of reality, realising our potential, improving the quality of our relationships and sharing our gifts and talents with the world. When you experience true happiness you have a deep sense of inner well-being, peace and vitality that doesn't dissipate in the face of life's inevitable challenges. When you experience true happiness you are no longer surviving life, but loving and living life fully. And I believe that this is the type of happiness we are all really trying to discover.

At this point you may be thinking 'I can't even achieve normal happiness!', 'That sounds too difficult for me' or even 'I don't understand!', but bear with me. Personally, I know that a few years ago I would have probably thought the idea of true happiness was possible for some people, but certainly not for me. It turns out I was wrong.

My search for happiness

For the last fifteen years, I have been exploring ways to find deeper fulfilment and happiness, not only for my patients but also for myself. This guide to happiness is the fruit of my search.

As a medical doctor I became aware, albeit after five years in practice, that a significant part of my drive to help others was rooted in my own need for healing. On the outside, I projected success and self-confidence; on the inside, however, I was fearful, insecure and unhappy. As the years went by, I became increasingly uncomfortable with the gap between what I was telling others to do and what I was failing to do for myself. My patients were getting better; I was getting worse. Unaddressed addictions, depression and low self-esteem eventually led to a crisis of identity and integrity, and I knew I could no longer go on living my life in the way that I was. I believe that many of us reach such moments.

The decision I made back then was to get honest and to do everything within my power to start creating a healthy, happy and fulfilling life for myself. The road since then has been long and challenging, but truly transformative. I am now blessed with an incredibly satisfying and rewarding life and I now walk my talk. What's more, my journey has revolutionised the way in which I work with my patients: rather than limiting myself to a conventional medical approach, I embrace the best of what works, be it from a nutritional, psychological or self-help angle. I also now understand that the art of medicine is not just about helping people recover from the symptoms of disease but, as importantly, to discover how to live a healthy and fulfilling life, and to do so in a way that restores a sense of wholeness, balance and inner joy.

Happiness can be yours too

This book is about making true happiness a reality in your own life. It doesn't matter if you are currently happy or depressed, experiencing a health problem or already enjoying a high level of health and vitality, true happiness is available to you, regardless of how you are right now, if you are willing to follow the advice in this book.

I wish you every success – a healthier, happier and more fulfilling life awaits you.

How to make this book work for you

I have structured this book in such a way as to keep what is potentially quite a complex subject as simple as possible. The following chapter, Choose Happiness Now, looks at what true happiness is and how it differs from 'normal' happiness. It features questionnaires that I use with my patients to assess where they stand in relation to the two most important factors that contribute to true happiness. Your answers to those questionnaires will give you a sense of where you are now and what is in store for you if you are willing to commit to nurturing and developing your happiness. Therefore, it is vital that you read it before moving on to the eight 'pillars' that are at the heart of my programme. (I refer to them as pillars simply because they are the fundamental building blocks for achieving true happiness.) The pillars are divided into three parts: The Essentials of Emotional Health and True Happiness, Overcoming Common Barriers to Emotional Health, and Maximise Your Happiness.

The essentials of emotional health and true happiness

Pillars One to Three form the foundation of my programme. Pillars One and Two provide you with what I consider to be some of the most effective ways to skilfully manage your thoughts and emotions. For example, in Pillar One, you will learn how to detach from 'negative' thoughts and discover how to loosen the hold that self-limiting beliefs have on you. Pillar Two will help you understand how you relate to your emotions and how you can 'process' them more skilfully. With these new tools under your belt, you are ready for Pillar Three – Live a Fulfilling and Meaningful Life – and the beginning of your journey to true happiness.

Overcoming common barriers to emotional health

Pillars Four to Six deal with the physical and psychological contributors to happiness and reveal how diet, lifestyle and a wide variety of different physical imbalances can impact on mood and emotional issues. Pillar Four will help you assess if you are meeting your body's needs for a nourishing diet, physical activity, sleep, rest, sunlight and a healthy environment, as these are all an essential part of experiencing health, vitality and happiness.

Pillar Five can be a revelation for some. The extent to which physical imbalances – such as those relating to neurotransmitters in the brain, blood sugar, allergies or hormones – affect our emotional health is often vastly underestimated. This pillar will help you identify if any of these factors are relevant to you. Other crucial barriers to happiness are those mental-health challenges that can arise at any point in our lives – stress, depression, anxiety and panic disorders, addictions, trauma and grief. Pillar Six will show you how to face such challenges.

Maximise your happiness

The final two pillars focus on compassionate self-acceptance and creating positive, healthy relationships. Pillar Seven acknowledges the fact that the failure to truly accept and embrace all of the different parts of our self is a major cause of suffering and unhappiness. In this pillar I show you simple and effective life-changing ways to increase your level of self-acceptance and self-love.

One of our deepest needs is to feel connected to others and have close, nourishing relationships. Pillar Eight is about creating those healthy relationships and mastering the skills to sustain them. While these two pillars are by far the most challenging, when embraced, they provide the gateway through which you can achieve your highest level of happiness.

While going through the pillars in sequence appears to be best for the majority of people that I work with, for others (and possibly for you), applying them in a way that meets your specific needs is also an option. The following case studies are quite different from one another, but they both demonstrate that should you decide to choose your own order, it is important to focus on no more than one or two pillars at a time, then move on when the time feels right.

CASE STUDY: KATHERINE

When Katherine first came to see me she was suffering from depression, anxiety and insomnia. Because she already had a mental-disease diagnosis (although of course the labels depression and anxiety tell us nothing about what is causing them), Katherine started to follow my suggestions in Pillar Six, identifying and addressing any mental-health challenges. After filling in the questionnaires it became apparent that trauma, passive anger and unprocessed grief were also affecting her mental health and restricting her enjoyment of life. Rather than working at an emotional–psychological level, however, Katherine chose to work at the physical level first. I helped her to identify her underlying physical imbalances (Pillar Five), which were related to the brain's neurotransmitters serotonin and GABA, blood-sugar imbalance and food intolerances. After addressing those, she went on to Pillar Four (Meet Your Physical Needs), focusing particularly on diet and sleep first.

Within two months Katherine was feeling much better, her sleep had improved and her depression had lifted, although she was still very much aware of background anxiety. I then supported her over a three-month period through Pillars One (Get Out of Your Head) and Two (Become a Master of Your Emotions). She loved the first pillar, and although she struggled to deal with her emotions in a more healthy and effective way initially, within three months she reported her anxiety as having gone. What's more, she had much higher energy levels than she had done for three years. With these positive foundations in place, she followed the suggestions in Pillar Three (Live a Fulfilling and Meaningful Life), focusing particularly on meeting emotional needs and gratitude. Three months later, she announced that she was ready to deal with her abuse from the past and the grief related to it (Pillar Six). Six months later, and after having taken part in a specialist workshop, Katherine said she was feeling the best she had ever felt.

CASE STUDY: FLORENCE

Florence was fit and well, and on a path of emotional and spiritual growth, but wanted guidance. Because she had no symptoms of mental illness and was meeting her physical needs pretty well, Florence started with Pillars One, Two and Three. After following their suggestions for three months, she moved on to Pillars Seven (Accept and Love Yourself) and Eight (Create Positive, Healthy Relationships), as she was keen to improve the level of emotional, physical and sexual intimacy that she and her partner of two years were experiencing.

After six months, Florence had made some significant changes – she now spent much more time on friendships and her relationship, and less on watching TV, cooking (which she had never enjoyed) and reading. Her level of connection with her partner blossomed and she started to teach basic gardening skills to children (this was a passion for her). She also reported a significant improvement in self-confidence and self-acceptance, and experienced a new lease of life and vitality.

Start a happiness chain reaction

Happiness often starts with one or two changes which, if successful, provide the energy, motivation and enthusiasm for making more. A typical example is Dave, who, because he was feeling sluggish and depressed, started his plan by implementing an exercise programme, coming off sugar, taking some supplements and practising gratitude. Within two weeks he was experiencing a much improved mood and better energy levels. He then decided to work through Pillar One, focusing particularly on defusing negative thoughts and mindfulness practice. After a month of that, he went on to Pillars Two and Three. Each step forward naturally flowed from the previous one.

Where should *you* start? My advice is to read through the book once, in order to get a feel for it. If you find yourself drawn to a particular pillar, I suggest you start with that one when you've finished reading all the pillars. If you aren't sure, then work through them in order, starting with Pillar One.

Before you begin

Before you start on your journey to true happiness, let me give you the same six pieces of advice that I give my patients before they start their programme.

1: Get committed and take action

If I had to summarise the key to discovering true happiness I would have to say it is this: committed daily action.

Many people who come to me for advice have good intentions and are excited at the prospect of changing their health, happiness and quality of life. However, within a few weeks (in some cases a few days), their motivation starts to waver and the action we agreed upon comes to a grinding stop. They then find themselves back where they started – only now they feel guilty, too. If this sounds familiar to you, try to focus on what you need to do *today*. When you catch your mind worrying about tomorrow or the future, bring it back to what needs to be done today.

I also have a lot of patients who don't experience this – or if they do, they take action to correct it. So, what's their secret? It's committed daily action. The challenge, of course, is that making changes to your life and the way you live and relate to it requires considerable effort, motivation, patience and perseverance – initially. You are essentially creating a new way of being, and to do this you need to be consistent in your new practices, skills and habits. There will be plenty of times when you will let things slip – it happens to all of us; the key, however, is to recommit to the journey when you notice this, and to re-instigate actions that will move you towards true happiness. The good news is that eventually, usually in just a few weeks or months, what was once hard-going (exercise, for example, or making time for intimate relationships) becomes much easier.

I often get asked how long it takes to implement all of the recommendations in my approach. Of course the answer is it depends on you, your circumstances, your willingness and your level of commitment. Most people that I work with experience a noticeable shift in the way they feel within days or weeks of adopting the recommendations in Pillar One. However, it can take much longer – possibly six to eighteen months – to implement everything you read in this book. Don't let that time-scale put you off! Remember, you're in this to transform your life and that doesn't happen with quick-fix solutions. The skills you will learn in this book are ones that you can – and should – continue to improve on throughout your life.

How to be and stay committed

Here are a few things that helped me, and subsequently my patients, to get and stay committed:

- Make a list of all of the benefits and positive consequences that will result from transforming your health and happiness. Add to your list over a period of days and even weeks. Look at your list at the start of each day and allow yourself to experience the feelings of excitement and empowerment that arise as you imagine yourself living this new life.

- Announce – to friends, family, partner, colleagues – your commitment to your plan, if doing so will be helpful. Enlist all the support you can get.

- Make a list of all of the potential barriers to implementing the suggestions in this book. Some common ones are not having enough time, low energy levels, being too busy, getting distracted easily, scepticism, tendency to self-sabotage and so on. Then, with a trusted friend (or life coach/therapist), write next to each one exactly what you can do to address it. For example, reduce amount of TV watched, get a personal trainer or rearrange your schedule.

- If you have any self-limiting beliefs – 'I am no good'; 'I can't change the way I am'; 'It's selfish to take time for myself' – take a look at the section on transforming beliefs in Pillar One (see page 30).

- Prior to going to bed each night, spend a couple of minutes mentally rehearsing the day ahead. Imagine yourself going through the day with a high level of happiness. The more accustomed your mind is to the idea of being this way, the easier it becomes.

- If the tasks and activities I recommend become a chore, find creative ways to revitalise them. For example, if you've been running on a treadmill at the gym but have started to get bored, consider enlisting the help of a personal trainer or varying your workout. The more flexible, creative and adaptable you are to your life, the easier it will become.

2: Have some emotional emergency tools to hand

Before my patients leave my clinic to start implementing their programme I teach them two emotional emergency tools that can be applied any time they feel overwhelmed or stressed. You'll find these very useful and if you consistently use either of them, I can guarantee that you will notice a reduction in your stress levels within a couple of days.

4/7 breathing

This is probably the simplest, yet one of the most effective, emotional emergency techniques.

- When you feel stressed, overwhelmed or tense, take a breath in to the count of four, then breathe out to the count of seven.

- Repeat this at least five times and notice how much better you feel.

- Breathing for a longer period of time on the out breath helps to calm the mind and increase the degree to which you relax. Try it out now.

Soften your gaze

Next time you are stressed about something, notice how narrow your focus of attention becomes. For example, you could be walking down a street and literally notice nothing around you. Now try this. Look slightly upwards, then, while continuing to look forward, soften your gaze so that you start to notice whatever is in the periphery of your vision – this defocusing instantly de-stresses both body and mind.

3: Identify and address any addictions

Be aware that if you have any untreated addictions you will not be able to fully benefit from the advice in this book. It is therefore essential that you address any addictions; otherwise they will sabotage your success in using this programme. Any recurring pattern of behaviour that is rooted in denial, dishonesty and/or secrecy and removes you from reality, responsibilities or relationships may indicate an underlying addiction. The most common addictions I see with my patients are addictions to work, busyness, alcohol, drugs, nicotine, prescribed medications, food, sex, relationships, gambling, shopping and misery. I recommend completing the questionnaire at http://www.s-p-q.com/ which measures some of these addictive tendencies. If the result is positive, please read the section on addictions on page 199.

4. Consider help and support

This is a self-help book, so it is designed to support you in your journey. But like any journey, it is best travelled with companions. For that reason, and because it will enhance your progress, if possible you should do this work with a friend – someone who is also committed to personal development and who is honest and able to listen to what you have to say. You might also want to consider signing up for my online True Happiness course or setting up a True Happiness study group (details are on my website www.discovertruehappiness.com). A study group can provide a wonderful way to evolve and grow within a community of like-minded people.

I also strongly encourage you, if you have any significant health issues such as addictions or a history of unresolved trauma, to work with a health professional who can provide you with personal support as you go through the book. If you want one-to-one support in implementing this programme you might want to consider working with one of my human potential coaches, who are trained in the True Happiness approach (see Resources, page 275).

5. Take a balanced approach to life

I call this taking the middle way. It's involves taking an honest look at how you live your life and making choices that will bring greater balance between being and doing, rest/relaxation and activity, and between quiet, personal time and social time. Living in the extreme keeps you out of balance and prevents you from moving forward. Regularly ask yourself the question, 'How I can simplify things and bring more balance into my life?'

6. Live with HEART

While each pillar involves undertaking specific actions, what underpins the success of my approach are the guiding principles represented by the acronym HEART. They are the threads that will guide you to true happiness. If you ever get overwhelmed, confused or stuck, remind yourself of the principles of HEART:

**H = Honesty, E = Emotional Awareness, A = Authenticity,
R = Responsibility, T = Trust**

Honesty

Honesty is first and foremost about having an honest relationship to reality, to 'what is'. It's about seeing through denial and acknowledging the reality about yourself, your life situation and your behaviour, past and present. Honesty is not for the faint-hearted. It requires courage and humility. Of course it will bring up all sorts of emotions – but once you have completed Pillar Two you will know how to manage and welcome these emotions. Another important – and very challenging – aspect of honesty is to be honest to our self about the intentions behind what we say and do. Are our words and actions motivated by truth, respect and love or lies, manipulation or control? Speaking only when your words and actions are motivated by truth, respect and love will rapidly accelerate your journey towards true happiness. A high level of honest sharing and expression is also a pre-requisite for trust and intimacy in relationships.

Emotional Awareness

Emotional awareness is the ability to be aware of, welcome and feel what you are feeling moment to moment. It's pretty challenging of course, but, like any skill, the more you practise it (Pillar Two shows you how), the easier it gets. Whenever you are stuck or unsure how to proceed with anything, turn your attention to what you are feeling and welcome it. This dissipates the suffering we experience when we deny and resist what we are feeling.

Authenticity

To be authentic is to be free from pretence and living in alignment with what I call your true self. It's about being aware of who you truly are, as opposed to who you think you are supposed to be. This is central to emotional health and happiness (I look at this in more detail in Pillar Seven). The more you trust the intuitive guidance of your true self, the quicker you will move towards true happiness.

Responsibility

This is about taking personal responsibility for the quality of your life experience as it is now. It requires you to acknowledge the fact that other people, events and experiences have had a significant influence on you in the past, but essentially you are now responsible for addressing the consequences of events and experiences – past and present. Taking 100 per cent responsibility for your feelings, needs and actions leads to a psychologically mature, blame-free way of living.

Trust

To trust is to let go of expectations and attachment to a specific outcome once you have done everything you can to make that outcome happen. Implicit in this is the truth that holding onto fixed expectations and outcomes is a sure way to increase your level of tension and suffering. If you have a tendency to be controlling, I'm sure you already know this. Trust is about finding a balance between taking action and letting go. If you want to throw a tennis ball to a friend, you have to pick it up in your hand, throw it and let go. If you don't do the letting go part, you and your friend are going to get very frustrated! And so it is with true happiness. You need to take the actions outlined in this book but, having taken those actions, let go of expectations. Trust, and focus on the process, not the goal. If that sounds difficult, don't worry – the guidance in Pillar One will help enormously.

Now you're ready to begin. Let's start by looking at the nature of happiness.

Choose happiness now

Why do you do what you do? What motivates you to be successful, have relationships, go to work, take up hobbies, spend time with friends or go on holiday? What is it that you are really looking for?

The answer given by at least 90 per cent of the people I ask is happiness. As William James, the father of modern-day psychology said, 'how to gain, how to keep, how to recover happiness, is in fact for most men at all times the secret motive of all they do'. Happiness turns out to be one of our deepest longings. Take Maria, for example. She came to me for help to overcome anxiety and low self-confidence so that she could perform better at work and develop a closer relationship with her partner. I asked her why she wanted these things and her answer was that she wanted to be happy and at peace. Put another way, Maria – like most people – wanted to experience less pain and suffering *and* more happiness and fulfilment.

Happiness matters

So why are so many of us seeking happiness? Well, the obvious answer is because it feels great. Think back to a time when you genuinely felt happy and at peace with yourself. As you recollect this time, notice how you feel lighter, more alive and how your life situation appears to be so much brighter and better.

Happiness also turns out to be one of the keys to good health. A nine-year Dutch study into the elderly, for example, found that those who were happy, optimistic or generally satisfied with life had around

50 per cent less risk of dying over the period of the study than those who were unhappy or pessimistic.[1] According to Professor Barbara Fredrickson, a psychologist and happiness researcher, when we feel happy we are also better able to broaden our capacity to engage more creatively and fully with life and build our potential for increased success on all levels. This includes at a physical, intellectual and social level.[2]

Essentially, happiness provides us with the 'fuel' to help us evolve, thrive and flourish. This is something I see consistently with my patients. I have learnt that the issues people present to me – the surface problems – are rarely the real issue. Yes, of course, physical illness, and such issues as depression, fear, stress and low self-esteem are distressing and can significantly reduce quality of life. But what I find time and time again, if I delve deeply, beyond the symptoms, is someone who wants happiness, fulfilment and love.

Of course, you can choose a conventional medical route and take medication to correct issues; this will alleviate the distressing symptoms, but – and again in my experience – the underlying need, the need for happiness, fulfilment and love, if not addressed will result in different problems arising. We should not kid ourselves that medication will solve the real problem. Take the case of George who took antidepressants to reduce his symptoms of depression and within two weeks starting getting back pain. Or Elaine, who treated her back pain with repeated visits to the chiropractor, then started to develop irritable bowel syndrome (IBS). Or Francis, who began to have anxiety and panic attacks a week after successfully eliminating her IBS symptoms with hypnotherapy.

If the failure to experience happiness is the problem, then the only lasting solution, as far as I am concerned, is to take the necessary action to discover the source of true happiness. If we don't 'hear' the story behind the symptoms, they will simply shift from one area to another and the true block to happiness will remain in place. For George, this was the loss of meaning and purpose that came with retirement; in Elaine's case, her back pain was related to the stuck grief over loss of her husband; and for Francis it was due to her constantly fighting reality (and an undiagnosed problem with addictions).

Are we getting any happier?

Sadly, despite considerable advances in overall standards of living and income, there has been no appreciable improvement in people's life satisfaction and happiness in the UK, US and many other countries in the last fifty years. Indeed, one poll found that the proportion of people saying they are very happy has fallen from 52 per cent in 1957 to just 36 per cent in 2005.[3] The World Health Organization reports that worldwide 121 million have depression and an estimated 5.8 per cent of men and 9.5 per cent of women experience a depressive episode in any given year.[4] The prevalence of depression is rising every year and it is now regarded, according to one report, as the world's most disabling disease – even more so than angina, asthma and diabetes.[5]

In a nutshell, many people are not very happy. What's more I also believe that many people who say they are happy, aren't truly happy. They are just good at sedating, avoiding and distracting themselves from their unhappiness. As a medical doctor and workshop leader I have seen how many of my patient's behaviours (and admittedly many of my own) are at their heart unskilled, misdirected strategies to avoid their unhappiness and emotional pain. These strategies and behaviours (which are explored more fully in Pillar Two) include blaming others, excessive busyness, overeating, compulsive judging of others and oneself, manipulation, lying, using food and sugar to change the way we feel, drinking alcohol, people pleasing, over-achieving, excessive TV watching, comparing, over-thinking, avoiding intimacy and overworking. Left unaddressed they increase our feelings of isolation, put us at risk of health problems, restrict our capacity for rich and satisfying relationships and stunt our emotional, psychological and spiritual growth. Essentially, we want happiness but we aren't experiencing it in a lasting way, because the choices we are making and strategies (behaviours) we are using are the wrong ones. But what exactly do we mean by happiness?

What is happiness?

At the most basic level, happiness is an umbrella term to describe a range of pleasant emotions that include contentment, pleasure, joy, enthusiasm, serenity and delight. Generally, when someone says they are happy they mean that they are satisfied with their life and that they are experiencing a preponderance of 'pleasant' emotions (and relatively few 'unpleasant' emotions). I refer to this type of happiness as 'normal' happiness.

As I pointed out briefly in the introduction, normal happiness is very much connected to what is going on in your life. If your relationships are going well, you have money in the bank, your health is good and you are successful at what you do, the chances are you will experience normal happiness. The clue that it's normal happiness is that it is conditional upon certain things being the way you want them to be. If you are made redundant unexpectedly or your partner is upset with you and your sense of happiness and well-being disappears, you know that the happiness you were experiencing was normal. The other hallmark of this type of happiness is that when we pursue it we often focus on short-term gains at the long-term expense of our health, relationships and personal growth; for example, working round the clock in pursuit of success and money, but neglecting our health and intimate relationships.

What is *true* happiness?

True happiness is worlds apart from normal happiness. Unlike normal happiness, which is dependent on what is happening in your life, true happiness is independent of what is happening. True happiness describes a deep sense of inner well-being, peace and vitality that is with you most of the time, in most circumstances. People who are truly happy typically experience a deep level of connection to themselves, other people and the natural world. They perceive everything as being alive and animated by an intelligent, benevolent life force. Their hearts are full of gratitude; they love life deeply. This is a difficult concept for many people – particularly when they are far from happy – but it is available to anyone who is willing to work on transforming their 'inner' life, as opposed to their outer circumstances. In fact, if you are committed to living with awareness, and living a life that is aligned with your deepest potential, then true happiness is inevitable.

So what is getting in the way?

When I ask in my workshops and lectures just what it is that's preventing us from experiencing our potential for true happiness, the answers are usually along the lines of time pressure, stress, lack of knowledge, information overload, perfectionism, keeping up with the Joneses, negative thinking, lack of role models, poor diet, mental illness, disease and so on. Of course, all of these can influence the way we feel and our mental health and well-being, but I believe there are two underlying factors that prevent many of us from experiencing our fullest potential for happiness and emotional health: the failure to emotionally and psychologically grow up and our failure to 'wake up' and live with greater awareness and acceptance of the present moment. Essentially, if we are to fulfil our potential for happiness, we must grow up and wake up. Much of the work in this book is designed to help you achieve this. Let me explain why.

The importance of growing up

Most of us who are essentially physically normal will, given a healthy environment and caregivers who are responsive and nurturing, evolve naturally into an adult who is emotionally mature. There is a strong creative, evolutionary instinct within us to do so. However, developmental psychologists believe that in the absence of an optimum loving environment, this maturation process doesn't happen. The majority of adults haven't completed this process and are, therefore, living, acting, thinking, feeling and relating as adolescents, rather than as mature adults.[6]

Think back to a time when you were arguing with someone, judging someone or using food to change the way you feel. How old did you feel in that moment? Quite often people will say I felt like a five-year-old, or a thirteen-year-old! Most of the time, when we when behave in this way, we have emotionally regressed. This is quite a revelation, but it goes a long way to explain why so many of us suffer unnecessarily and, in turn, create so much suffering for others, society and even the planet. We are simply not functioning as emotionally mature adults on a consistent basis. Instead, we are allowing our immature ego to dictate the way we live.

Say hello to your ego

Most of us spend a great deal of our time identified with and operating from our ego. What is the ego? It's a bundle of thoughts, beliefs, emotions, conditioning and fear-based desires and needs. The ego is the 'I' that we identify with and take ourselves to be. However, it's important to recognise that there are two versions of the ego – the emotionally immature and the emotionally mature ego. In order to understand the process of growing up, let's take a look at each.

The emotionally immature ego

This version of the ego is focused on what it can get *from* life. When we are identified with and living from an emotionally immature ego, our thoughts and actions are driven by the emotion of fear and two associated core beliefs: 'I don't have enough' and 'I am not enough'. As a result, we tend to be self-centred and focused on getting and acquiring 'things' in order to feel as comfortable and safe as possible. The list in the box below provides some of the most common indicators that our emotionally immature ego is in charge of our life. You will probably find you have some of these characteristics but don't worry, that's common. The point is to acknowledge that this is so and to realise that operating from your emotionally immature ego is preventing you from fulfilling your potential and experiencing true happiness. The purpose of this book is to help you change that by revealing how to evolve and 'mature' your ego.

INDICATORS OF LOW/MODERATE MATURITY

- Fighting, avoiding and resisting reality

- Tending to avoid anything that has the potential to cause discomfort

- Wanting to be right, wanting to be special

- Not being aware of what you are feeling and/or finding it difficult to share what you are feeling with others

- Focusing on feeling good and avoiding pain/discomfort

- Taking most things personally

- Struggling to experience emotional intimacy and/or having a history of multiple relationship breakdowns

- Giving to others in order to get something from them

- Feeling stuck in your life

- Not proactively addressing addictive behaviours or mental ill health

- Blaming others for the way you feel

- Excessive amounts of comparing, defensiveness, worry and judgement (of self and others)

- The need for immediate gratification

- Controlling or sedating your feelings with alcohol, caffeine, sugar and food, perfectionism, drugs, excessive busyness or compulsive working, TV, gossip, controlling and manipulating others

- Emotionally over-reacting or under-reacting to various situations and people

- Having little or no awareness of your values

The emotionally mature ego

The second version of the ego is the emotionally mature ego. Someone with a healthy, mature ego has a high level of self-acceptance, they take responsibility for their life situation, they take good care of their health, they are committed to fulfilling (or realising) their potential and they treat others as equals and with respect. Their focus is very much on how they can contribute *to* life.

In this book I am going to outline everything you need to do to evolve into your emotionally mature self. While this will enrich your life and improve your health considerably, by itself it's not enough to help you achieve true happiness. For true happiness you also need to wake up.

Waking up to the present

Have you ever walked away from someone with whom you were speaking and realised that you didn't actually hear a word they said? Or do you sometimes eat something and then can't recall what it tasted like? If so, and I'm guessing you answered yes to both of these, where were you? In both instances your body was present to the experience but your awareness was caught up in your thoughts. Your mind and body were in two different places – they were out of sync.

Contrast those experiences with a time in which you were completely immersed in the moment, caught up in the flow of your experience – for example, it might have been when you were skiing or running, making love, watching a sunset or seeing something of great beauty. Really think about that time, take a couple of deep breaths and allow those feelings to get stronger inside of you – notice how much calmer, peaceful and powerful you feel. In these instances your body and mind are present to the same experience – they are aligned with the present moment. This alignment of our awareness with our experience in the moment is called present-moment awareness.

Present-moment awareness is a state of being awake, alert and in alignment with the each moment as it is. Rather than avoiding reality – which includes what we are thinking and feeling – present-moment awareness is a way of inhabiting our experience (internal and external) with awareness and without filtering or creating a story about our experience.

We spend the majority of our mental time in a state of mind in which we are either avoiding reality or just simply not aware of what is going on because we are so caught up in our thoughts and feelings. Of course that's OK for some of the time, we do need to reflect on the past and future, analyse our situation and contemplate our experiences – that's a highly useful thing to do and one of the gifts of the human mind. But getting caught up in our thoughts and feelings or resisting reality is not good for us.

Resisting reality creates suffering

Resistance to 'what is' creates suffering and unhappiness. The reason for this is that the root cause of most tension and suffering (there are exceptions) is our continual struggle with reality: most of us have a hard time letting our experience be as it is. By judging, rejecting, controlling and sedating certain areas of our experience that cause us discomfort or pain, for example by ignoring the anxiety we might be feeling in our body when we are with someone, we protect and maintain our state of balance and normality but we also progressively become disconnected from our true self. By avoiding and withdrawing our awareness from these painful or uncomfortable aspects of ourselves, we cut ourselves off from our true self – the source of true happiness.

Waking up involves living with greater awareness and acceptance of the present moment. This doesn't mean we have to necessarily *like* the present moment – but accept the reality that it is happening. By accepting the reality of each moment, rather than fighting and resisting it, we open ourselves to the experience of life and our true self. (In Pillars One and Two I'll show you how to develop present-moment awareness.)

THE TRUE SELF

The true self is the rarely accessed part of us that embraces all of the different parts of ourself, including ego, while simultaneously transcending them all. The true self:

- Knows how to get in touch with and realise our fullest potential

- Is experienced as a deep sense of well-being, vitality and peace of mind

- Knows the perfect response to each unfolding moment

- Is the source of creativity and intuition

- Provides us with clarity, insight, guidance and natural confidence

Pillar Seven explores the true self in more depth. All you need to know for now is that the true self lies beyond your thoughts, emotions and ego.

How grown up and awake are you?

As a starting point on your journey to true happiness, complete the following questionnaires to assess how emotionally mature and aware of the present moment you are. Be mindful of your inner critic using your results to judge that you *should* be more grown up or more 'awake'. The purpose is to clearly see and accept the reality of where you are at, so that you can now move forward with greater clarity and motivation.

QUESTIONNAIRE: Emotional maturity

Below are twenty statements with which you may agree or disagree. Using the scale below, indicate the extent to which you agree with each item by choosing the appropriate number. Be as open and honest in your response as possible, and don't get too tangled up in the exact meaning of the statements – just trust your instinct.

strongly agree = 7, agree = 6, slightly agree = 5
neither agree nor disagree = 4, slightly disagree = 3, disagree = 2,
strongly disagree = 1

I am:

- Actively creating a healthy, meaningful and fulfilling life that is directed by my values – the things that are most important to me ☐

- Committed to realising my full potential ☐

- Engaging in rich and satisfying relationships ☐

- Committed to being the most loving person I can be ☐

- Approaching life with the attitude of 'what can I give', rather than 'what can I get' ☐

- Able to give to/help others without any conditions or expectations most of the time ☐

- True to myself and the needs of the situation I am in most of the time ☐

- Actively embracing healthy self-care ☐

- Proactively addressing my blocks to emotional, physical and sexual intimacy ☐

- Moving through the emotions that are preventing me from making peace with the past. I'm releasing my resentments as and when I am aware of them ☐

- Working with my thoughts and emotions in a way that promotes greater health and personal growth ☐

- Facing reality wherever possible and taking appropriate actions when relevant and appropriate ☐

- Able to adapt flexibly and creatively to situations and to embrace change ☐

- Working towards compassionate acceptance of myself and others ☐

- Able to truly listen to others and experience empathy ☐

- Embracing change ☐

- Enjoying my life, having fun and experiencing a light-heartedness most of the time ☐

- Able to have and maintain healthy physical, sexual, emotional, intellectual and spiritual boundaries with others ☐

- Actively addressing any addictions, health problems, mental health or trauma issues that I have ☐

- Able to communicate clearly and respectfully my needs and perspectives to others ☐

Total score ☐

Interpreting your score

A score of 120 or more indicates that you have a high level of emotional maturity. Congratulations! You are probably at peace with yourself and thriving and flourishing as a mature adult. You can use this book to fine-tune any areas that are currently imbalanced and take your happiness level even higher.

A **score between 80 and 119** indicates that you presently have a moderate level of emotional maturity. Most people who fall into this category usually have a history of using self-help approaches, and/or were brought up by caregivers who were (most of the time) able to provide the affection, attention, support and love that they needed as children. While life might be going OK for you, you still have a lot of potential to fulfil. Following and implementing the suggestions in this book will take you to a whole new level of happiness.

A **score less than 80** indicates that you currently have a low level of emotional maturity. (See page 6, which highlights some of the many indicators that typify someone with a low or moderate level of emotional maturity.) Your score suggests that you are surviving, rather than thriving in life. It's unlikely that you have ever been taught the skills to manage your emotions and create healthy relationships. What's more, you are probably carrying a lot of unprocessed emotions and possible trauma from the past that is holding you back. However, the fact you are reading this book means that while your journey to true happiness will be challenging, you have the potential to transform completely the quality of your life if you are willing to follow my suggestions. You are where I once was, as well as many of my patients. But I promise you that by making some changes to the way you live life, you can know true happiness and real fulfilment.

QUESTIONNAIRE: Present-moment awareness

Below are twenty statements with which you may agree or disagree. Using the scale below, indicate the extent to which you agree with each item by choosing the appropriate number. Be as open and honest in your response as possible. Again, don't get caught up in the exact meaning of the statements, just trust your instinct.

strongly agree = 7, agree = 6, slightly agree = 5
neither agree nor disagree = 4, slightly disagree = 3, disagree = 2,
strongly disagree = 1

I am:

- Always fully present in the moment ☐
- Open to and welcoming all experiences as they occur ☐
- Experiencing an undercurrent of gratefulness throughout my waking moments ☐
- Aware of what I am thinking, feeling and sensing in the moment with ease ☐
- Aware of a strong ongoing feeling of vitality within my body ☐
- Aware of a natural sense of well-being, peace and joy that is unaffected by my emotions and thoughts ☐
- Able to control and direct my attention away from negative thoughts/images at will ☐
- Responding to challenging situations from awareness and from what I intuitively feel is right ☐
- Present and aware when eating ☐
- Welcoming all emotions equally ☐
- Trusting that I will know what to do or how to respond when challenged by my life circumstances ☐
- Embracing the realisation that fulfilment exists right here, right now ☐
- Able to know without doubt that when I maliciously hurt others I hurt myself ☐
- Able to be present to the person I am with, irrespective of what they say or do ☐
- Actively embracing not knowing ☐
- Wholeheartedly engaging life with awareness and acceptance ☐
- Waking up to the realisation that consciousness (life) is evolving through me ☐

- Responding to my life situation with actions that are creative, spontaneous and unconditioned ☐

- Not focused on becoming somebody but committed to remembering who I am ☐

- Living with the knowledge that everything is an invitation to wake up to my true nature ☐

Total score ☐

Interpreting your score

A score of 120 or more indicates that you have a high level of present-moment awareness. You are experiencing the joy of being and living in alignment with your true self. You can, however, use this book to fine-tune any areas that are currently imbalanced and take your happiness level even higher.

A score between 80 and 119 indicates that you presently are able to experience present-moment awareness from time to time and in some circumstances. While life might be going OK for you, you still have a lot of potential yet to be fulfilled. Following and implementing the suggestions in this book will take you to a whole new level of happiness.

A score less than 80 indicates that you currently have a low level of present-moment awareness. Your score suggests that you would benefit considerably from learning how to become more present – the pillars that are particularly relevant to you are Pillar One (Get Out of Your Head) and Pillar Two (Become a Master of Your Emotions).

The 14-day happiness test

The previous questionnaires will have given you a good idea of where you stand with regard to how emotionally mature and awake you are, but if you're interested in taking this a bit further and discovering how truly happy you are, I highly recommend you take my 14-day Happiness Test, which you'll find in the appendix. It is challenging, as it requires you to give up the strategies you use to control or sedate your feelings – for example, alcohol, caffeine, overworking, watching too much TV – but it will get to the heart of how happy you are.

Summary

- The majority of people are not very happy and a significant number of those who say they are, aren't truly happy. They are just good at sedating, avoiding and distracting themselves from their unhappiness.

- Most individuals focus on creating 'normal' happiness. This type of happiness is dependent on certain conditions being met and fulfilled. The person who pursues normal happiness does so in a way that often limits their potential for emotional or spiritual growth.

- True happiness, in contrast, is not dependent on outer circumstances and describes a deep sense of inner well-being, peace and vitality that is with you most of the time, in most circumstances.

- In order to experience true happiness we need to grow up and wake up. Growing up involves taking actions that will enable your ego to evolve emotionally and become more healthy and balanced. Waking up involves living with greater awareness and acceptance of the present moment. By accepting the reality of each moment, rather than fighting and resisting it, we open ourselves to the experience of life and our true self.

Now you're ready to begin. Good luck with your journey!

Part One

The essentials of emotional health and happiness

Pillar One: Get out of your head

You are useless.

What feelings and thoughts has that three-word sentence triggered in you? Do you have an uncomfortable feeling in your body? Do you notice any tension? Has it 'rattled your cage' or are you feeling perfectly happy and at peace? This might not have been a particularly pleasant way to start, but I wanted to demonstrate to you these important formulas for unhappiness and happiness:

> Believing/identifying with any
> negative thought, word or image   = unhappiness

> Not believing/not identifying with
> a negative thought, word or image   = happiness

You choose happiness

In any given moment you choose your level of happiness according to the way you relate to what you are thinking. If you believe your thoughts and identify with them – you are at one, or 'fused', with them – they will determine how you feel. So, if you have a positive, life-enhancing thought, such as 'Isn't life great!' and you are fused to it, positive feelings will be triggered and you will feel good. If your thought is 'I am useless', however, and you are fused to it, unpleasant feelings will be triggered within you.

When you are fused to your thoughts, you are at their mercy – you become a victim of your own thinking, as they have control and power over you. But by not allowing your thoughts to hold you to ransom and by changing your relationship with them from one that is adversarial to one that is accepting and light-hearted you transform the way you feel – often quickly.

Thoughts are not reality

Most thoughts do not accurately reflect reality. In fact the majority of thoughts that you have originate from past experiences and are therefore nothing more or less than distortions of present-moment reality. Put another way, most thoughts are tainted with the past and distortions of the truth.

What's more, thoughts are not powerful, although they may appear to be so. Their power is related to the degree that we attach to them and infuse them with our attention, belief and emotion. It's us, for better or worse, who make thoughts powerful. Being controlled by thoughts is therefore an illusion; what's really happening is that we are giving our power to the thoughts. They are simply impersonal sparks of information and perspective flying through your awareness that you can choose to engage with if you wish. The key word here is *choose*. In any given moment you have the ability (with a little bit of training) to select which thoughts you attach to and believe.

Given that most thoughts are not reality, one of the most important things you can do, in each and every moment, is to not believe the negative story or thoughts created by your mind. Why? Because it is so easy – and so common – to become stuck in a cycle of negative thoughts and emotions and this hampers our ability to experience our true self, the source of true happiness.

How thoughts relate to your feelings

For quite some time, the phrase 'thoughts create our feelings' (or 'feelings follow thoughts') has been in vogue. In fact, this isn't true.

Psychologists Joe Griffin and Ivan Tyrell developed a theory, the APET model, that helps to explain the relationship between thoughts and feelings.[7] I think it's important and very helpful to understand this because it makes sense of why so many of us get stuck in a vicious cycle of thinking and feeling. I call this the unhappiness cycle.

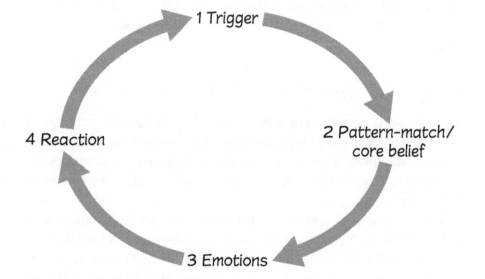

The unhappiness cycle

Most of us spend our time pedalling around the unhappiness cycle – a self-perpetuating cycle from which our apparent choices and decisions originate, though, as you'll discover, they are distorted by our past experiences and by our self-limiting beliefs. The unhappiness cycle has four components:

1. Trigger
This refers to the thought you are having or the situation, circumstance or event outside of you. It's whatever gets your attention.

2. Pattern-match
The event, situation or thought is then cross-referenced against similar past events for comparison. It is as if we ask ourselves, 'Does this match something I am expecting to happen or some previous experience?' Most commonly, it's compared to the memory of an experience from the past – embedded within which is a self-limiting

belief, or core belief, (such as, 'I am not good enough') and the residual (unprocessed) emotional charge relating to it.

3. Emotions

If a situation triggers a memory (or memories) of something similar that happened in the past, the emotions tagged to it will arise in the body as feelings and sensations. For example, you might feel anxious and notice tension in your solar plexus area. The clue that the emotional charge has more to do with the past than the present is that your emotional response is disproportionately strong for the situation.

4. Reaction

This is what automatically happens in response to your feelings, in order to change what you are feeling. For example, you might start getting negative thoughts (thoughts therefore come after feelings), start arguing back, shut down emotionally, reach for some comfort food or take your stress out on someone or something related. The new thoughts now act like triggers and start the cycle again.

At first glance, this might seem a little complicated, but it's worth reading through it a couple of times so that you really get it. You will see that unless there is an intervention at any one of the four levels, the system is effectively on auto-pilot – there is no conscious decision-making in there at all.

Let me give you an example. Marjorie, a forty-three-year-old woman with stress-related illness and chronic lower-back pain, shared with me a thought that was causing her a lot of distress. She told me, 'My husband is selfish; he doesn't love me.' This thought was her trigger (1). Next, her mind automatically cross-referenced the thought with similar situations from her past. And guess what? She found one. Her father had been emotionally and physically absent for most of her childhood and the conclusion she had come to, as a child, was that he didn't love her (2 – pattern match). With this came a lot of anger and emotional pain which she felt as heaviness in her chest and throat. The bulk of the intensity of the pain did not relate to her husband (although some did), but to her father (3 – emotions). In response to the pain, she used some common passive–aggressive anger strategies, such as remaining distant and aloof from her husband and criticising him. On top of that, she had further distressing thoughts as to how she was going get her own back (4 – reaction). In a nutshell, Marjorie was trapped in the unhappiness cycle and couldn't get out of it.

How to exit the unhappiness cycle

While the unhappiness cycle demonstrates how we can get stuck, it does also reveal how to get out of the rut and into happiness. The first thing I taught Marjorie was to notice any time she was unhappy and to say to herself, 'I am stuck in an unhappiness cycle.' Next, I taught her how to defuse from her distressing thought (the trigger – stage 1), which you will learn about below. Looking at the diagram, you can see that by doing this, stage 2 is then not activated. The cycle is broken. We also did some work on her beliefs and used a process called Conscious Regression (see page 30) to stop the transference of anger relating to Marjorie's father on to her husband.

To get you started and to help you develop the ability to stand back and watch your thoughts, I recommend the practice of mindfulness. Once you have developed a degree of mindfulness you will find it much easier to defuse your negative thoughts.

Practise mindfulness

There are many different definitions of mindfulness. I use the term to describe an alert, calm presence with what is. Being mindful means bringing an attitude of openness, curiosity and acceptance to the reality of whatever you are noticing. Mindfulness training has emerged as a powerful, evidence-based tool for enhancing psychological health. It is empirically supported as an effective intervention in a wide range of clinical disorders, including chronic pain, anxiety disorders, depression, PTSD, OCD, substance abuse and borderline personality disorder. One study at University of Wales and John D. Teasdale at the Medical Research Council in England found that eight weekly sessions of mindfulness halved the rate of relapse in people with three or more episodes of depression.[8] Although mindfulness has only recently been embraced by Western psychology, it is an ancient practice found in a wide range of Eastern philosophies, including Buddhism, Taoism and yoga.

Getting started

I highly recommend that you set aside some time each day to practise mindfulness. The following exercise and the suggestions for life awareness practices have proved popular with my patients. I suggest you start with breath awareness.

EXERCISE: Breath awareness

Breath awareness involves noticing and following the breath without any analysis, control or judgement. It is at the heart of many different meditation practices and is the foundation of present-moment awareness. Curiously, by observing and experiencing the breath, without any intention of changing it, the breath will often automatically slow down and naturally become fuller. You should allocate about 10 to 20 minutes for this exercise.

- Sit comfortably on the floor or in a chair.

- Close your eyes and bring your awareness to an aspect of your breathing. You may choose to focus your attention on the passage of air in and out of your nostrils, the rising and falling of your chest or the movement of your belly as you breathe in and out. Just choose one and stick with it throughout the session.

- Don't do anything with the breath; don't try to control it in any way, just allow it to be – just observe it.

- Notice how your mind wanders. This will happen and it's completely OK, it's part of the process. Notice the story that your mind is telling you, for example 'I can't do this', 'this is boring' and so on. Don't engage with or fight the story, just gently return your attention back to the breath.

- Stay relaxed and keep observing, moment by moment, the movements of the breath. When you get caught up in thinking, again, just gently return your attention to your breath.

So it's a very simple exercise, but one that can be quite challenging given the fact that most of us are so used to getting caught up in the stream of our thoughts and feelings. The real key is to be gentle with yourself and to be persistent, no matter what. Although you might feel disheartened initially because of the mind's propensity to pull you out of present-moment awareness, by being playful with this exercise, keeping it light (not being overtly tense or serious about it) and adopting an attitude of curiosity (you are exploring what awareness feels like) you should make good progress and soon start to feel more calm and less 'engaged' with your thoughts.

Life awareness practices

As the name suggests, this involves bringing awareness to whatever you are doing as you are doing it. Although everything offers an opportunity to practise awareness, I have found that bringing mindfulness to the experience of eating and walking has been a very useful tool for increasing present-moment awareness. When you do the following try to bring an attitude of openness and curiosity. So for example:

- Next time you go for a walk, rather than going up into your head to think, notice five things you can see (without labelling them and thinking about them), then gently turn your attention to five things you hear and then to five things you can feel (for example the ground underfoot, the wind against your face). Keep rotating around your senses and allow yourself to become present to them.

- Most of us eat unconsciously; that is we eat without necessarily being aware of the experience of eating as we eat. Next time you eat something, really slow down the process of eating and allow yourself to engage the process of eating mindfully. Look at the food, smell it, chew it slowly and taste it fully. Become aware of how your body is feeling as you eat the food. Is it increasing or decreasing your energy levels? Does it feel healthy or unhealthy? Is it supporting your health or taking away from your health? Once you get used to mindful eating, you start to get a real sense of what the food is going to do to your body and health.

There are numerous other ways to learn the skill of mindfulness. There are many excellent books and CDs on it and, even better, mindfulness training courses. These usually last for eight weeks and are becoming increasingly widely available. See Resources, page 281 for further guidance.

MEDITATION

Meditation is a very popular form of mind training. The focus is usually on training your attention and discovering who you are beyond thoughts and emotions, i.e. discovering your true self. However, rather than a technique to be practised, I regard meditation more as a way of being that enables you to wake up and live life consciously and deliberately. People who meditate regularly experience improvements in their creativity, present-moment awareness, physical health (especially the immune system) and happiness, as well as reduced stress, anxiety and depression.[9] While most meditation approaches involve being still, I am a big fan of movement meditation practices such as Movement Medicine and Five Rhythms. I recommend you check them out, especially if being still is not something that comes easily to you. I also have a tip for you, one that really helped my own meditation practice and that of the meditation group I run. Before you meditate, just say to yourself 'I am no-mind' and notice how that shifts your experience. Most people meditate with what I call the controlling mind. Unfortunately, it's the wrong part to meditate with! Pillar Seven explores this in more detail.

Defuse your 'negative' thoughts

Defusing negative thoughts is the process that I taught Marjorie and one that I have used successfully with many of my patients. If you are committed to your emotional health, it is an essential skill. I am not asking you to suppress or replace the negative thought with a more positive one, because a positive thought is still only a thought – a distortion of reality. In fact, one study found that people who suppress personally relevant intrusive thoughts (the type often seen in obsessive compulsive disorder) experience more intrusive thoughts and more distress than those who are willing to accept the reality of their thoughts.[10]

Techniques for defusing negative thoughts

The intention behind these techniques is not to control, change or get rid of unpleasant thoughts, but to reclaim your energy and attention from them. A positive shift in the way you feel is often the result.

So any time you become aware of a negative or unpleasant thought or image, reclaim your power from it: take a couple of long, slow, deep breaths and then use one of the following techniques:

- Repeat the thought out loud very slowly three or four times, allowing a gap of at least five seconds between each word. This is my favourite defusion technique because it allows awareness to arise as you do it. Notice how much more calm you feel as you do this.

- Say to yourself, 'My head is telling a story that . . . '

- Witness and observe your thoughts without judging them (see the Breath Awareness exercise on page 23).

- Imagine those thoughts are coming from a small gremlin and say to yourself, 'I sense and accept you.' This is a particularly good one if you have a strong inner critic or are prone to judging others.

More often than not, using any one of these will reduce the intensity of the uncomfortable feelings that you are experiencing. It's often just a case of finding the one that works for you. Over the next few days, experiment with them to find out which works. Note the following advice, however:

- If you are experiencing a lot of strong emotion that is keeping you trapped in the thought, do your 4/7 breathing (see page xxiii), then use one of the emotional processing tools in Pillar Two (see pages 52–60).

- If the negative thoughts are recurring, you might need to address any underlying physical imbalances (Pillar Five) or mental-health challenges (Pillar Six) or the underlying beliefs (see page 30) that are contributing to them.

One of the concerns that some of my patients have is that by disengaging negative thoughts they are potentially ignoring a situation that is a real problem. The truth is, in fact, the opposite. Acknowledging and accepting the reality of the thought, and then disengaging from it, creates space for awareness and your true self to provide you with direction or insight – if that is required.

Take Sophie, for example – a twenty-four-year-old receptionist who was experiencing anxiety. One of the troubling thoughts that was triggering a lot of unhappiness was that she might lose her job because her company was being restructured. I explained to Sophie that this was not actually a negative thought, because it did accurately reflect the reality that her company was making redundancies. However, what *was* negative was that Sophie was fused with that thought, and, as a result, she was allowing that thought to trigger a whole range of other distressing thoughts: 'They don't want me', 'I am not going to be able to afford my mortgage' or 'I don't know what to do', for example. These thoughts, in turn, triggered anxiety within her.

Sophie used the defusion techniques with great success and, after following my suggestions in Pillars Two and Three over a period of two months, she was able to completely relieve her symptoms and start creating a more fulfilling life for herself.

Other tips for dealing with 'negative' thoughts

When you get caught up in a negative thought, ask yourself one of the following questions and notice how it shifts your energy:

- Will this matter in ten years from now?

- I wonder what I can do to access peace of mind right now?

- What lesson do I have to learn? This last question is very important. I believe that we can learn and grow from every experience. By asking this question we shift our relationship with the situation from problem to opportunity.

Investigate your thinking

One of the most useful tools that I have come across to help individuals break out of the unhappiness cycle is 'The Work'.[11] Developed by the spiritual teacher Byron Katie, The Work is designed to identify and investigate the thoughts that trigger pain, suffering and distress. This takes defusion to the next level, as it not only encourages you to disengage the negative thought, but it also guides you through a process in which insight and positive shifts in perspective are often brought about.

The basis of The Work is the understanding that our most intimate relationship is with our own thoughts, and that the way we relate to them significantly influences the way we feel, react and behave. Because most of us believe and identify with our thoughts without questioning them, they wield considerable power over us. However, if we question and investigate them using this process of enquiry, not only is it possible to reduce the negative hold they have over us, but we can also bring about a significant shift in clarity and understanding. It's not about changing your thoughts but changing your *relationship* to them.

One of the many enlightening realisations that emerges in using The Work is that, often, things we think about in relation to other people are things that are often about ourselves. The exercise below gives you a flavour of The Work but I also recommend that you look at Byron Katie's book or website (see Resources, page 280).

A taste of The Work

Next time you have a distressing or limiting thought about yourself or your partner, such as, 'He doesn't want to be with me', try the following. Part of the process is writing your answers down. And it doesn't matter if they're petty and childish – that's helpful.

1. Ask yourself, 'Is this true?' Usually the immediate response is 'Yes' 'No'.

2. Now ask yourself, 'Can I absolutely know that it is true?' This time, don't rush to answer. Breathe deeply and allow an honest answer

to rise in your awareness. Whatever answer you get is fine. If you answer 'No', notice how this shifts the energy in your body.

3. Ask yourself, 'What happens when I believe that thought?' How do you react? What happens? Be specific and detailed. This gives you some insight into the power and limiting influence that this thought currently has over your life.

4. Now ask yourself, 'Who would I be without this thought?' Notice the impact that this has on the way you feel and how it changes the way you would react to your partner. Give yourself plenty of time to become aware of the new feelings that arise. Breathe deeply and give them plenty of space to come up. Having done this, the real key is the turnaround, which is a way of experiencing the opposite of what you believe to be true.

5. In the turnaround you are turning around the concept, idea or thought that you are working with. You turn it in three directions – to the opposite, to the other and to yourself. You then ask yourself: 'Is this as true or more true than the original statement?' For example, 'Paul should love me' is changed to:

- Paul should *not* love me.

- I should love Paul.

- I should love myself.

6. Finally, write a statement in which you are willing to embrace reality, because it is fighting or resisting the reality that is at the heart of suffering. For example, your statement might be: 'I am willing to experience moments when Paul is not loving to me.'

Notice how freeing this is. By completing this final step, my patient not only embraced reality – because of course there will be times when Paul is not loving to his wife – but discovered that the real so-called problem was that she wasn't loving herself. She couldn't control Paul – he was who he was – but she could control and influence the relationship she had to herself. As a result, she started to redirect her energy and attention away from Paul and focused on taking care of and cultivating more respect for herself. This exercise took her just fifteen minutes, but provided one of the most invaluable insights of her life to date.

The six steps above allow you to shift the power and attention from the thought to awareness, to separate yourself progressively from the thought, so that you can decide yourself what is true for you.

Transform any self-limiting beliefs

In the unhappiness cycle on page 20, you learnt that many of your emotions and 'negative' thoughts originate from past experiences and the beliefs built into them. Learning how to transform these underlying beliefs is an important part of creating a high level of emotional health.

Beliefs are the silent assumptions that you hold about what is good, what is bad, how you should and should not be and how others should and should not be. They provide the set of rules by which you live and the conviction (which are emotionally supercharged beliefs) that when you live in alignment with these beliefs you will be comfortable and when you do something that is out of alignment with your beliefs you will experience discomfort and resistance. The problem is not so much that beliefs exist – we all need beliefs because they tell us what is most important and meaningful for us – but that they remain unexamined. Put simply, if you are not aware of them, then they, for better or worse, are in charge of you.

There are two ways I work with my patients' beliefs. The first involves something called conscious regression; the second is the book of beliefs.

Conscious regression

Conscious regression is an invaluable tool for resolving the root beliefs and emotional charges from which negative thoughts and emotions emerge. Because it can bring up strong emotions, only use it if you feel it is safe and right to do so. If you are unsure, and especially if you have a history of significant trauma, I suggest you read the section on trauma in Pillar Six, page 202.

Next time you get emotionally triggered – especially when it is disproportionate to the situation – take your attention off the person or situation and do the following:

- Notice what you are thinking – for example, 'He shouldn't be so loud'.

- Notice what you are feeling – for example, 'I am feeling angry'.

- Identify the judgement – for example, 'He should be quiet'.

- Now, think of another time when you had a similar feeling or response.

- Keep going back in time until you discover the earliest memory of when you felt the same way. (If you feel uncertain about doing this or if you are feeling overwhelmed, you should stop and seek the support of a health professional.)

- Notice what you are feeling and sensing in your body. What would you have liked to have done or said (if it was guaranteed there would be no negative repercussions)? Say those things now, imagining that you are there right now. If you need to scream or shout, use a pillow over your mouth or twist a towel. Allow the energy to come out of you. Alternatively use EmoTrance (see page 53) to process what you are feeling.

- Now identify where that judgement came from – this is usually from your caregivers (for example, 'My mother always said being loud is not good').

- Again, notice what you are feeling and sensing in your body. Now process it, as indicated above, until you feel energised and at peace.

The purpose of this exercise is to help illuminate and then start to address many of the beliefs that are rooted in the past. The present, when filtered through the beliefs of the past, prevents us from experiencing the fullness of now. As you apply this exercise regularly, you will find that you will become much less reactive to situations and that judgements will start to decrease quite considerably.

Illuminate your book of beliefs

Each of us has a book of beliefs, a virtual book containing details of how and who we should and should not be in the world. This book of beliefs provides the template and standards against which we measure and judge ourselves and others. The problem for most people is that the considerable majority of beliefs, like our thoughts, are not true; they are borrowed from other people and are significantly restricting their ability to enjoy freedom and fulfilment.

What's more, we each have an inner critic, an aspect of our personality that is constantly scrutinising how we live up to our beliefs (rules). If I have a belief that I should be rich and successful and I am not, then my inner critic will start to give me a hard time: 'Why am I so useless?', 'I need to do better' and so on. While the intention of the inner critic is to help me achieve those beliefs, in the belief that doing so will bring me happiness and fulfilment, the reality is that it doesn't. It just brings stress and inner tension. The alternative is to take a look at the book of beliefs and to decide for ourselves which ones we do and do not want – to choose those that will bring us greater happiness and fulfilment and to ditch the others.

Using your book of beliefs

For each of the following categories (and any others you want to cover), write down the rules that come to mind – all of your shoulds and shouldn'ts: body, sex, mind, emotions, relationships, masculinity or femininity, success, money, morals, other people and spirituality. Many of your rules will seem ridiculous, but write them down none the less. Claire, a workshop participant, listed her shoulds and shouldn'ts relating to her body as: my body ought to be perfect; I should not have cellulite; my breasts should be bigger; I should be taller; my skin should be fairer; I should be able to run quicker.

At one level, of course, it's OK to have aspirations – not having cellulite, for example. However, fighting the reality that you have cellulite will only lead to emotional distress, tension and pain. The key is in accepting reality, then taking action to address the issue from a place of acceptance. (This is covered in detail in Pillar Seven.) Here are two other options for working with your beliefs.

A very simple way to reduce the impact of a belief on the way you think, act feel and behave is to say it very slowly. I mentioned this earlier on in the thought-defusion section (see page 26). I use this a lot when working with patients and it works really well. Essentially, saying it slowly drains away the emotional intensity attached to the thought and allows a sense of awareness and 'spaciousness' to arise in between and around each thought. As you become aware of this you realise – and this can be quite a revelation – that the stressful thoughts are simply thoughts, not reality.

Another effective and liberating way to work with beliefs is through the use of Byron Katie's The Work, which we touched upon earlier. Focusing on one belief at a time, you bring the four questions and turnaround questions to that belief – doing this brings about a sense of freedom from the belief. (To help you with this, you can download the free 'one-belief-at-a-time' worksheet from Byron Katie's website.)

Other suggestions include:

- Observe without judgement every time you notice a should or should-not statement arising in your thinking. If it helps, just say to yourself: 'Oh there's my inner critic telling me what I should and should not do.'

- Acknowledge your fears and share/talk about them with a friend.

- Process your fears/feelings fully using Cradling or EmoTrance (see Pillar Two).

PILLAR ONE: Summary

- Believing and 'fusing' with negative thoughts causes suffering and unhappiness.

- Thoughts are not reality.

- Most thoughts are more about the past than the present.

- By disengaging your thinking, you open up to your true self – your inner source of joy, love and peace.

- You always have a choice as to whether you believe a thought or not.

- Most negative thoughts about others will reveal an insight about yourself when investigated.

Pillar Two: Become a master of your emotions

Do you deliberately avoid or control certain emotions, such as anger, fear or sadness? Do you find yourself emotionally overreacting to situations? Do you feel uncomfortable or tense around people who are expressing sadness or anger? If your answer is 'Yes' to any of these questions, you are not alone.

Few of us have been taught how to experience, feel and manage our emotions in a way that promotes optimal health, healing, intimacy and personal growth. This is the essence of good emotional health but many of us don't possess, or have never been given, the knowledge, skills and tools for managing our emotions. This is not surprising, given that we live in an emotion-phobic society; one in which the head rules, not the heart. And the reality is that many of us compulsively avoid, sedate or control certain emotions without realising that in so doing we limit our capacity for happiness and true intimacy with others.

CASE STUDY: JULIAN

Julian was a successful self-employed business owner who drove a £100,000 car, lived in a seven-bedroom mansion and had his own private plane. At a financial level, he was doing really well, but not so well emotionally. His reason for coming to see me was that he was prone to uncontrolled bursts of anger, in which he would 'lose the plot'. This was putting a considerable strain on his relationships with his wife, who had already threatened to leave him, and his employees, many of whom were fearful around him. Like many people with this sort of problem, Julian's anger wasn't really about other people and events – they were just the triggers. It was very much more to do with the residual emotions surrounding a traumatic, abusive childhood and the fact that he hadn't learnt how to manage his anger in a healthy, mature way. His unresolved past was coming back to haunt him in the present.

Julian was a pleasure to work with because of his willingness to learn and to try my suggestions. I taught him many of the emotional-management approaches that I am about to share with you and, in parallel, he had a series of breathwork sessions to help process and integrate the residual emotions relating to the past. Breathwork (which is covered later on in this pillar) is, in my experience, an effective way to transform emotional blocks. After six months, Julian's anger outbursts had stopped and he was 'more at peace with himself than he had ever been'.

I believe that the adversarial relationship that most people, like Julian, have with their emotions is a significant contributing factor to their unhappiness. Almost without exception, every patient or workshop attendee that I have ever met is knowingly or unknowingly engaged in an ongoing battle with their emotions. If you are to improve your emotional health it's vital that you learn to welcome all emotions and respond to them in a positive way – this is at the heart of true happiness. Before we look at how you can do that, let's examine the nature of emotions.

What are emotions?

People have a lot of different ideas about what emotions are. Personally, I find it useful to think of emotions as simply being energy in motion; currents and patterns of energy that are experienced as sensations moving through the body in response to the mind (thoughts, beliefs, images and memories) and to the functioning of the physical body. Only once they have been engaged with thoughts and 'labelled' do these energy patterns become emotions such as fear, sadness, happiness and so on.

What is the purpose of emotions?

Emotions are information. They are messages telling you what is happening in your body and mind and whether you are meeting their needs. For optimum health and well-being your body needs to have healthy food, rest, sleep, relaxation, physical activity, water, warmth and shelter. It also needs to be relatively free from a variety of body-related problems, such as imbalances of hormones, neurotransmitters (chemicals that communicate mood) and nutrients, as well as allergies, inflammation and toxicity. If these needs aren't being met, your body will communicate it to you through distressing emotions like irritability and sadness.

You also have emotional needs which include the need for security, giving and receiving positive attention, connection with the wider community, an intimate close relationship with at least one other person, autonomy, status, competence, privacy, meaning and purpose. If these aren't being met, your emotions will tell you. For example, if I am not meeting my need for friendship, I might experience sadness or loneliness; and if I don't feel competent in what I do, I might experience embarrassment, fear and nervousness. By listening to your emotions, you will often discover an unmet need which, when met, will result in the emotion disappearing. Once an emotion has served its purpose it no longer needs to be there.

THE RELATIONSHIP BETWEEN STRONG EMOTIONAL REACTIONS AND THE PAST

Have you ever overreacted to a situation and felt emotions that were disproportionate with what was warranted? Or have you witnessed yourself automatically and predictably reacting to a situation, just like you've done a hundred times before? We've all had moments when we've been surprised and sometimes shocked by what's come out of us, or surprised at how the way someone looked at us or said something could trigger such a strong emotional response. Why is this?

It's called pattern matching and it's happening all of the time.[12] Your brain has built-in pattern-matching technology. It is a very clever survival and learning mechanism that loosely compares your current experience (including events going on around you and your own thoughts and images) to similar past experiences. At one level, it's very helpful, as it allows you, for example, to get inside a car and know, without having to think about it, how to drive.

There is, however, a significant downside to the process of pattern matching, one that can cause significant distress and stop you from learning and growing through experiences. For example, if you grew up in a household where your mother or father criticised you (the past), part of you will automatically be primed to look for any evidence of being criticised by those around you now (the present). So, if your partner says something that you interpret as having even the slightest hint of criticism, the event will be pattern-matched, and you will immediately feel the emotional load from the past (anger/frustration) arising inside of you. Because this process is so quick and automatic, it's easy to see why you would attribute the way you feel to your situation, whereas, in truth, your situation has simply reawakened the past. This is part of the process outlined in the unhappiness cycle in Pillar One (see page 20).

Why are emotions so important?

Although emotions tend to be undervalued by some therapists and avoided or controlled by many people, they are actually at the heart of what it means to live a healthy and fulfilling life. Emotions provide richness, texture and depth to your life experience and a bridge across which you can deepen your connection to yourself, to others and to the natural world. If you just had thoughts without emotions, you would live a dry and independent existence without a sense of fun, community or love.

What's more, emotions serve an evolutionary purpose; they are an integral part of your in-built survival and self-preservation system. For example, the emotion of fear will trigger responses in the body that enable it to fight, flee or freeze, while feelings of love will help to ensure that you remain connected and bonded to others, which, in turn, increases your chances of survival.

Emotions are also linked to higher functions that include healing, achievement and spiritual growth. I have observed with my patients how there is an intelligence within people that brings unacknowledged emotions into awareness in order for them to be dealt with (i.e. processed and integrated). When these are ignored or unprocessed they just recycle themselves as physical or emotional symptoms. In contrast, when they are processed, positive shifts in health and the healing process often take place.

Another function of emotions is to provide the fuel, energy and motivation to help you take action to achieve your goals, which, in turn, brings a sense of meaning and purpose. Emotions, being information, communicate to you what you need and what is needed in this moment at a deeper level than thought. Recognising this and acting on it will help you to nurture and take better care of yourself.

Are there negative emotions?

One of the most common misunderstandings concerning emotions is the idea that certain emotions are negative or positive. This is understandable, particularly if you are living life on the basis of normal happiness, whereby you focus on minimising the experience of uncomfortable 'negative' emotions (fear, anger and sadness) and maximising your experience of comfortable, pleasurable ones (joy and elation). This polarisation of emotions is unfortunate, because they all contribute to the experience of being human. Negating any of these emotions disconnects us from a valuable source of insight and information. Emotions are not inherently bad. What determines whether they are healthy or unhealthy is our relationship to them – our emotional-management style.

Assess your emotional-management style

The way you deal with and manage your emotions is what determines whether they have a positive or detrimental impact on your health, life and relationships. You are now going to discover your emotional-management style. Although you might use a few emotions, depending on the situation and how you are feeling at the time, one style tends to dominate – it's that one that I want you to identify. If, having done this, your mind starts to judge you, resist engaging with those judgements. The purpose of this assessment is to show you what a mature, healthy emotional-management style looks like and to help you see where you are right now.

The mature style

Someone who has a mature emotional-management style:

- Understands that emotions are information and is able to welcome the full range of emotions fully without needing to change, control or sedate them

- Does not label emotions good or bad, but regards them simply as movements of energy

- Knows how to express and use their emotions in ways that are appropriate to the situation

- Is more understanding of other people when they are experiencing emotions and will allow them to move through their emotions rather than closing them down

- Knows how to take care of themselves if they do experience strong emotions – for example, by calling a friend or using an emotional-processing tool (the ones I recommend to my patients are included later in this pillar)

The open style

Someone who has an open emotional-management style:

- Understands that emotions are an invaluable part of being human

- Will allow themselves to experience their emotions (for instance, anger or sadness), but unlike those who use a proactive approach, they are more likely to identify with their emotion and wait for the emotion to pass

- Will tolerate other people being emotional, but not necessarily be comfortable with the situation and will experience some degree of resistance

The closed style

Someone who has a closed emotional-management style:

- Keeps their so-called negative emotions, for instance anger, sadness or fear, hidden, because they are uncomfortable with them

- May or may not be aware of what they are feeling

- Tends to fuse (identify) with their emotions and thoughts

- Will be fearful of expressing emotions, because, commonly, they have a fear of being criticised, losing control, being weak (if they believe that showing emotion is a sign of weakness) or upsetting others

- Will find it difficult to experience intimacy and connection because they struggle to reveal and share their inner experience

- Will be upset, intimidated and/or overwhelmed by those who do show their emotions

- Will tend to project their emotions on to others; for example, falsely accusing someone of being angry, when the truth is that they are angry themselves

- Will probably use food, alcohol, smoking, drugs, work, sex, gambling and so on to control and sedate their emotions

- Will dismiss others who are emotional, perhaps by saying, 'You really shouldn't be upset', 'It's not that bad', 'Look on the bright side' and so on

The anti-emotion style

Someone who has an anti-emotion emotional-management style:

- Will either reveal very little emotion or be blown hot and cold by their emotions – there is no healthy middle ground

- Is for the majority of time fused (identified) with their emotions and thoughts

- Responds to other people's 'negative' emotions with hostility; for example, a mother might say to her child, 'If you don't stop crying I'll give you something to cry about' or, 'You can stop that now you ungrateful little so and so'

- Is constantly involved in power struggles and only knows how to 'feel in control' by putting other people down

- Is emotionally unstable and unpredictable, which can be very intimidating for people close to them

- Will probably use food, alcohol, smoking, drugs, work, sex, gambling and so on to control and sedate their emotions

Having read through these descriptions you can probably guess that the healthiest way to manage emotions is the mature one, followed by the open approach, closed approach and then the anti-emotion approach. The good news is that these are not fixed levels, so if your dominant way of managing emotions is one of the latter three, that just indicates the potential for you to 'grow up' and develop a more mature approach by using skills you will learn in this pillar.

Identify your emotional-control strategies

In order to get in touch with your emotions so that you can relate to and work with them in a more healthy way, one of the first – and potentially very challenging – tasks is to illuminate the ways in which you sedate, control and distract yourself from your emotions. Most of these strategies – emotional suppression, use of alcohol, food and drugs, projection and being overly positive or optimistic, for example – are deeply ingrained habits, which means it can be quite hard, initially, to see when you are using them. (One of the best ways to uncover how you use them is to do my 14-day Happiness Test – see the Appendix, page 267.)

When do emotional-control strategies become problematic?

Control methods are not intrinsically bad or negative; they are simply ways in which you protect yourself from experiencing pain and discomfort. Using a chocolate bar to create pleasurable feelings when you are feeling tired or bored, for example, is OK as long as it is used only occasionally and you are taking action to resolve the underlying issues. You are only human after all. They do, however, become a problem when they are used excessively, inappropriately, illegally, as a means of avoiding reality, relationships and responsibilities and as an alternative to emotional processing. So, control methods become difficult if:

- You rely on them to the extent that they create problems of their own; for example, you distract yourself from work that needs to be completed by watching excessive amounts of TV

- You use them for too long and they become automatic habits, preventing you from being in touch with reality – your true thoughts and feelings

- They consume your energy, which could otherwise be directed towards life-enhancing growth and activities

- You live life in resistance to or avoidance of reality; this not only creates stress, but also makes for an inauthentic life

- They prevent you from meeting certain needs; for example, avoidance of intimate relationships because of an underlying fear of being abandoned or overwhelmed will prevent you from meeting the need for closeness and intimacy

- You deny and fail to embrace and integrate part of yourself, accumulate emotional pain, reduce your experience of aliveness and restrict your potential for emotional growth and creativity

- They contribute to health problems; for example, excessive consumption of cakes and chocolates can lead to excessive weight gain and poor health

- They prevent you from focusing on activities that you value; if, for example you have a love of singing, but you have a fear of humiliation and therefore stop singing

- They are used in situations that can't work; for example, drowning your sorrows in alcohol for weeks and months after becoming unemployed, rather than seeking support and using emotion-processing tools to help yourself

Research has found that while avoiding uncomfortable thoughts and feelings might provide some relief in the short term, the intensity of the pain and discomfort and the frequency with which you experience them often increases in the long term.[13] Also, the ability to control your emotions goes down, anxiety levels go up and the feeling of being out of control rises with it. Studies have linked anxiety, panic attacks, obsessive compulsive disorder (OCD), phobias and depression to the avoidance of certain thoughts and emotions.[14] For example, someone who has low self-confidence, coupled with feelings of inadequacy when in social situations, might say they are unavailable to go out with their friends in order to reduce those feelings. While this strategy might decrease their discomfort in the short term, it will increase their overall pain and discomfort in the long term, because they are not meeting their emotional need for attention and community, nor are they living life in alignment with what they value – in this case, friendship.

So the good news is that by learning how to work with your thoughts and emotions – and not against them – you can reduce considerably the amount of stress and tension that you experience. Before you can do this, however, you need to understand how you avoid your emotions.

The most common emotional-control strategies

Here are some of the most common emotional-control strategies. You might need to read through them a couple of times and keep referring back to assess which ones you use.

Denial
Denial occurs when a person is faced with a fact that is too uncomfortable to accept and rejects it, insisting that it is not true, despite what may be overwhelming evidence. Other forms of denial include

denial by lying, either by telling outright lies or by leaving out certain details; denial of responsibility by blaming, minimising or justifying (this works by re-directing attention away from oneself); and denial of impact, in which a person refuses to reflect on the consequences of their actions.

Projection

This happens when we project onto and assign to another individual, the feelings, thoughts and traits (positive and negative) that we find unacceptable within ourselves. For example, asking your partner why they are so angry, when in fact it is you who is angry.

Transference

This is an unconscious mechanism that gets played out in most relationships. It happens when we relate to another person as though they were our parents or a significant other from the past. In doing so we experience feelings, expectations and beliefs about the person we are with, that are actually related to past relationships. We literally enter a time warp. Transference results in a distorted view of the person present and, unless resolved, prevents us from truly seeing them as they are.

Displacement

This involves directing feelings relating to one person, onto another person. The classic example of this is shouting and getting angry at your children a couple of hours after your boss embarrassed you in a meeting. The angry feelings really belong with your boss, but they were displaced onto the children, because you were unable to process or contain them effectively at the time they arose.

Suppression

This involves deliberately pushing away certain thoughts and feelings. Suppression is associated with high levels of control, both in terms of the amount of feeling and which feelings you allow yourself to experience and also to express. Most people who suppress their emotions engage a lot of energy in maintaining the pretence of being calm and composed.

Withdrawal

This involves avoiding certain situations, people and interactions in order to steer clear of the uncomfortable feelings they trigger inside you. A patient of mine avoided social situations as far as possible because of his feelings of vulnerability and shame, and a fear of being laughed at.

Self-criticism

This involves speaking to yourself in a harsh and direct way in order to change the way you feel. Favourite phrases of the inner critic are, 'You are pathetic' or 'What an idiot.' While some people think that self-criticism is important in order to achieve things and prevent themselves from making mistakes, self-criticism – as we will explore later, see page 183 – only adds to emotional pain and low self-esteem.

Positive thinking

This uses positive self-talk as a means to eradicate negative thoughts and feelings: 'I am strong, confident and capable' or 'Stay focused and calm'. Positive self-talk does have its place and can be effective; for example, I recommend positive affirmations to my patients that are then linked into taking positive action. More often than not, however, it is used to avoid reality which, in turn, prevents the release of wisdom and insight from the emotion that is being experienced.

Sedation

This happens any time that you use something to calm and soothe your emotions, most commonly alcohol, food, prescribed medications and drugs, such as cannabis. Rather than making the emotions go away, however, they simply reduce your awareness of them.

Fantasy

This involves escaping into an inner imaginary world. While creative imagination is useful and positive, if fantasy is used to escape reality then it is a control method.

Disassociation

This takes place when you withdraw your awareness from your body and emotions, so that you are not aware of what you are feeling. It happens automatically and can be an indicator of a past history of trauma, although not necessarily so.

While this may seem like a long list already, there are many other emotional-control strategies. These include keeping busy and distracted, changing the subject, watching TV, arguing, getting angry, fighting, getting physically and/or emotionally abusive, shouting, blaming others, hurting oneself, depriving oneself, smoking, going to sleep, worrying, over-analysing, changing your thoughts, complaining to others, talking excessively, reading, surfing the Internet, having/pursuing sexual encounters, planning revenge and so on.

What are your emotional-control strategies?

On a piece of paper or in a journal, write down a list of all the ways in which you try to control your emotions. Give yourself plenty of time to do this. Next to each of the strategies you identify, write their long-term negative consequences – this is the really important part of the exercise.

So, someone may write, for example:

Behaviour	Eating to avoid feelings of sadness and shame
Consequences	8kg overweight, reduced self-confidence, criticism from partner
Behaviour:	Arguing when I feel hurt and vulnerable
Consequences:	Distance between me and my partner, reduced emotional intimacy
Behaviour:	Worrying when I feel scared and anxious
Consequences:	Reduced quality of sleep; being distracted and unable to focus on my work

Once you've finished this list, take a couple of moments to reread it. The purpose of this exercise is to illuminate the fact that while your avoidance strategies may alleviate some of your pain and upset in the short term, they often have negative consequences in the long term. I will show you more positive strategies later, in the final part of this pillar. Most of my patients find it very helpful to discuss their findings with their partner, a friend, therapist or True Happiness support group. I encourage you to do the same.

Increase your emotional-body awareness

Once you start to disengage your emotional-avoidance control strategies the next task is to deliberately bring your awareness and attention into your body. The reason for this is that the body is where the emotions are located. However, I don't mean the physical body, I'm referring to the emotional body. Knowing about the emotional body is essential to understanding emotional health. Increasing numbers of doctors, especially those with a holistic orientation, are starting to appreciate the importance of improving the health of the physical and emotional body in parallel.

The emotional body – our 'second' body

We know without any shadow of a doubt that we have a physical body because we can see it and touch it. The emotional body is different because it can't be seen (although some individuals claim to be able to see it), but it can be felt and sensed.

In contrast to the physical body, which is made of atoms and molecules, the emotional body is much more subtle, it's made of energy and vibration. It's an energy field that permeates and influences the physical body and yet is separate from the body. As I pointed out earlier, emotions are simply movements of energy within the emotional body – they are energy in motion. This is not groundbreaking news. All of the traditional cultures recognise the existence and importance of this energy or life force. In China, for example, it's referred to as 'qi' and in India 'prana'. Restoring the harmonious flow of energy through the emotional body is regarded as one of the keys to optimum health and vitality, and many complementary and alternative healing approaches, from acupuncture and hands-on healing to yoga and qigong, attempt to do this. While some conventional medical doctors and scientists balk at the idea, my own personal and professional experience has been that these approaches are often of great benefit. For that reason, I recommend my patients explore them if they are drawn to do so.

For those patients who are looking to improve their emotional health (and the majority want to or need to), I encourage them to work actively on developing emotional-body awareness – the capacity to be aware of the movements of energy (emotion) within their body in each and every moment – on the premise and reassurance that I will also teach them how to deal with the emotions that will inevitably arise when they do so.

There are many ways to bring your awareness and attention into your body; it's a case of finding a couple of ways that work for you. Suggestions include sensual and non-sensual physical touch, physical exercise, yoga, Pilates, qigong and bodywork, especially massage and rolfing. My personal favourite is yoga nidra, an ancient yogic process of meditation that enables you to enter a profound state of relaxation, while remaining totally alert and present. In addition to this, I have found the daily practice of the following emotional-body awareness exercise to be invaluable. What's more, developing your level of emotional awareness will really enhance the benefit you experience from the emotional processing tools that I recommend later, particularly EmoTrance.

EXERCISE: Emotional-body awareness

This takes a couple of minutes to do and can be done pretty much anywhere and at any time. To start off with, however, I suggest that you do it at home, either while sitting comfortably or lying down. For the first couple of weeks, I recommend using it at least two or three times a day.

- Take a couple of deep breaths, close your eyes and focus your attention inside your physical body. As you continue to breathe, scan from head to toe and as you do so notice the aliveness within your body. Where is that sense of aliveness and tingling located in your body? Is it in your feet, legs, abdomen, chest, head, hands or arms?

- When you find it, be with it and feel it – enjoy what you are feeling. If your mind distracts you, simply bring your attention back to what you are feeling. Maybe you can feel this aliveness in many areas – if so, great, feel those together. Notice as you continue doing this that the feelings of aliveness increase. The aliveness that you are now aware of – don't worry if you can't feel much, it gets easier the more you practise – is your emotional body.

So, what's the point of this exercise? Well, firstly, you will probably feel much more calm, grounded and centred having done it. Secondly, with time and practice, you will be quicker to notice bodily sensations and emotions that are communicating to you, whether they are emotions, hunger, tension or tiredness. By being aware of them, you will then be able to work with and manage them more effectively. It will also make it easier to process emotions using the tools outlined later in this pillar.

Improve your emotional literacy

Emotional literacy refers to your ability to identify and describe what you are feeling – and to do so in a way that is simple, direct and non-judgemental, and which keeps the focus on you. This is quite complex, particularly if you have a tendency to point the finger of blame at others or if you have limited emotional awareness.

However, the good news is that emotional literacy is a skill that can be learnt and often picked up within a few days and weeks. Not only is it at the heart of effective communication and emotional intimacy, but by getting in touch with what you are feeling, you will know whether your emotional needs are being met or not. Realising that you are feeling irritable, for example, will alert you to the fact that one (or more) of your emotional needs is not being met – say, the need to be heard. What's more, naming a feeling – by saying, 'I feel sad', for example – helps to direct your attention to what you are feeling and, in doing so, makes it much easier to then shift out of your head and feel (process) that feeling.

When I work with patients who have limited emotional-body awareness or who struggle to *feel* their feelings, I get them to practise labelling their feelings first, then to drop the label and just feel what they are feeling.

How to improve your emotional literacy

For the next twenty-four hours, practise identifying your feelings to yourself by using the four basic feelings: 'I feel sad', 'I feel bad', 'I feel mad' (angry) and 'I feel glad'. This might sound pretty basic, but it will get you off to a great start.

Label your feelings

As you get used to using mad, bad, sad or glad, dig a little deeper to see if you can find a word that resonates with what you are feeling; when you get the right word, you will probably feel a positive shift of energy in your body. Once you have got used to identifying whatever it is you are feeling, the next step is to process them using the suggestions in the next section, page 51.

Unpleasant feelings

These include feeling tense, anxious, stressed, agitated, perturbed, shocked, unsettled, irritable, nervous, depressed, unhappy, despondent, bereaved, hurt, lonely, miserable, regretful, vulnerable, fragile, sensitive, hesitant, envious, jealous, pining, tired, sleepy, lethargic, weary, embarrassed, ashamed, mortified, disconnected, detached, withdrawn, afraid, panicked, scared, worried, wary, annoyed, aggravated, impatient, irritable, frustrated, angry, resentful, enraged, appalled, horrified, ambivalent, confused, hesitant and bewildered.

Pleasant feelings

These include happy, delighted, joyful, amused, peaceful, calm, contented, fulfilled, relaxed, still, rejuvenated, refreshed, hopeful, encouraged, grateful, moved, touched, thankful, thrilled, elated, exhilarated, excited, enthusiastic, astonished, loving, compassionate, open-hearted, confident, proud, interested, curious, amazed and inspired.

Become skilful in emotional processing

So what is a healthy way to deal with emotions? Early on in this pillar you started to shine light on the different ways in which you try to avoid and sedate your emotions. These strategies were learnt early on in life, and they represented your best effort at trying to minimise the experience of uncomfortable emotions so that you could get on with life.

But what would happen if you replaced your old (immature) strategies with new (mature) ones which, when used, actually moved you towards greater health, intimacy and true happiness. What if it was possible to address the underlying causes of any emotional discomfort so that you no longer needed to run away from or fight your feelings? What if the key to happiness and fulfilment was to not focus exclusively on doing things that make you feel good, but to train yourself to get good at feeling?

How emotions are processed

Hopefully, having read the previous sections, you're now aware of how you avoid emotions and are becoming more aware of them. Remember that emotions are basically information. In order to receive that information, we need to welcome our emotions, accept them, digest them and then, depending on the situation, either use the information to make a decision or take action or, if the emotion relates to the past, process it. The emotional processing tools that follow will help you do that. First let me explain how the body processes emotions.

Built into the same intelligence or body wisdom that co-ordinates the trillions of interactions of your body–mind is a system for processing emotions. (By body–mind I simply mean the mind and body seen as two aspects of the same entity rather than as separate.) All of us, to differing degrees, experience stress, hurt, disappointment and sadness, so it makes sense that nature should provide us with a way of absorbing, digesting and processing emotions. Our emotional-processing system is essentially a form of emotional housekeeping.

One important way in which we process emotion was discovered by Joe Griffin, a founder member of an organisation called the Human Givens Institute (see page 18). In a nutshell, they propose that when you experience emotional arousal during the day (for example, if you worry about money or a relationship problem), but are unable to resolve it in some way (process it), the charge will be deactivated by the process of dreaming. The incomplete emotional arousals are discharged and completed through the often bizarre and exaggerated scenarios acted out in your dreams. However, this requires longer periods of REM (rapid eye movement) sleep and the amount of deep, restorative sleep experienced is, therefore, significantly shortened. So, you wake in the morning feeling exhausted, with less energy and motivation to take action and take care of your emotional and physical needs, and you are more likely to put a negative spin on your circumstances. The vicious cycle continues.[15]

Tools for emotional processing

Although there are many ways to deal with emotions (most of which involve control and sedation of emotion), when it comes to improving your emotional health and discovering true happiness the focus really needs to be on processing/digesting the emotion. The main emotional processing skills that I use and teach, in addition to simply allowing yourself to feel fully your emotions, are:

> EmoTrance
> Cradling
> Honest self-expression

I suggest that you experiment with each of these in order to discover which works best for you. You might, for example, use different skills depending on the situation and emotion you are working with. Although it might initially feel clumsy or uncomfortable using them, with patience and practice they will eventually become second nature. (I also use Breathwork, see page 56, which is highly effective but it needs to be learned from a practitioner.)

I often get asked what one should do when strong feelings, such as anger, arise in the moment, but there isn't the time or it's an inappropriate place to address them. You have a number of options. I suggest using 4/7 breathing (page xxiii) to bring you into the present moment and then later on in the day check in with yourself to see if you are carrying any strong emotions. Alternatively, as you get more proficient in using the tools that follow, you can use them in the moment without anyone noticing (EmoTrance is particularly good in this situation).

EmoTrance

EmoTrance is a simple and highly effective emotional processing tool that I teach most of my patients. It is based on the idea that a healthy state of mind and body arises when subtle energy (qi) flows without interruption through and out of the body. When we hold on to, suppress or repress an emotional upset this stops the energy from flowing, which in turn leads to distressing mental and sometimes physical symptoms. EmoTrance is designed to restore the flow of energy through the emotional body that I mentioned earlier on.

EXERCISE: How to use EmoTrance

Give yourself at least 20 minutes to do this at a time when you know you won't be disturbed. Using this tool might at first appear to be a bit tricky, but once you've tried it a couple of times you'll see how straightforward it is.

1. Think of a statement, fact, thought or criticism that causes you to feel upset or to feel 'negative' emotions. This could be a person or a phrase that upsets you, such as 'You're fat,' 'You're useless,' or 'You disappoint me'.

2. Write this issue down on a piece of paper, turn it face down, take a deep breath, then turn it back over and allow yourself to feel any emotions. (If you don't feel anything, choose another issue.)

3. Pay close attention to where you feel it in your body. If there is more than one site, choose the one that feels strongest. What you are feeling is just trapped energy or emotion that wants to move.

4. If you can, gently place your hands on that area and get a sense of

the direction in which the energy wants to go. If you don't get an immediate indication, start massaging the area with your hands, continuing to concentrate on softening the energy as you do so.

5. When the energy starts to move, which it will do, get a feel for which part of your body it wants to exit through. This can be any location – top of the head, mouth, nose, hands, feet, anything goes! If it's not obvious which exit route it wants to take, just be patient and continue softening until it starts exiting your body.

6. Allow all the energy to exit your body. If it appears to get 'stuck', gently rub that area or trace the route you feel it wants to take with one of your hands, as that often helps.

7. More often than not, there will be residual energy in your body, so to make sure that all of the emotional charge has been de-activated, repeat the whole procedure again, starting from number 3.

8. Keep repeating until you feel no unpleasant sensation at all. On average it takes two to three cycles. If you feel lighter, more ener-gised and much clearer around the issue, then you have success-fully deactivated that emotional upset – well done!

9. Take a moment to consider how this experience will change your behaviour and the way you feel about the issue.

The key with this exercise is to be patient with yourself. Part of your mind will try to rush you and convince you that it isn't working for you. If this happens to you, just slow down, breathe deeply and con-tinue.

In summary, when you have an emotionally charged issue to work with:

- Locate where you are feeling the energy

- Tell it to soften and flow

- Get a sense of where it wants to exit your body

- Allow it to flow, and if you catch yourself trying to force it or getting frustrated by it, breathe deeply and let go

- Repeat until you have gone as far as you can

See Resources, page 280, for recommended resources relating to Emo-Trance.

Cradling

This is a tool that I have personally found to be very useful when it comes to managing my own emotions. Many of my patients have also really benefited from it. In a nutshell it involves noticing, meeting, greeting and cradling your emotions with warmth and affection. It sounds complicated, but in practice it's pretty straightforward. To make it easier I have divided it into three stages.

EXERCISE: How to use Cradling

The first stage involves gently *noticing* and *observing* the fact that there is an emotion (energy) arising within you and that it is associated with a variety of bodily sensations.

- Just notice and observe the bodily sensation. I recommend, especially if you are new to this, to start by also identifying and labelling your emotion, for example 'I am feeling fearful', and then having done so, return your awareness to the emotion and its associated bodily sensations.

Stage two involves *meeting* and *greeting* that emotion. Stage one was about observing at a distance the emotion, now you are moving towards it, making contact with it and feeling it.

- Keep breathing gently; keep your attention on what you are feeling – if it helps, focus on and breath into the area where the emotions/bodily sensations are strongest.

Stage three involves *cradling* your emotions. What do I mean by that? It means feeling what you are feeling but with the same affection and warmth that a loving adult would cuddle a child who was upset. When cradling your emotions you are accepting and embracing them just as they are.

- With awareness and warmth, gently 'enter' the emotion. This can be challenging, particularly if you are used to sedating or controlling your emotions, but I promise you, as with any new skill, the more you practise it the easier it becomes. Stay with your emotions until you experience the shift to spaciousness and lightness. This can happen in a few seconds to minutes or sometimes longer – 5 to 10 minutes – but it almost always does happen. Give it all the time it needs and keep your focus on feeling rather than rushing it or trying to get to the peacefulness on the other side – even though it is tempting to do that!

While the goal of this exercise is simply to feel and cradle your emotions, the consequence of doing so is the lightness, spaciousness and sense of peace that opens up. What's more, it is often followed by a positive shift in perspective. The issue that was troubling you before now feels different; you are more at peace with it and are now able to embrace a mature stance.

BREATHWORK

An effective and direct way to process and integrate suppressed and repressed emotions is through the practice of conscious connected breathing. Unlike most breathing techniques, which allow a pause between the out-breath and the in-breath, conscious connected breathing involves breathing without any gap or break between the two. Doing so allows the subconscious mind to bring into your awareness any emotional material that needs integrating. Welcoming and breathing through the emotions that arise results in their integration, which often leads to the experience of transcendent peace and even bliss. It is very powerful healing work and an approach that I recommend to patients who are carrying a significant amount of unprocessed pain in their emotional body. However, breathwork needs to be learnt from an experienced practitioner. See Resources, page 280, for more information.

Honest self-expression

One of the simplest ways to process feelings is to share what you are feeling with another person in a way that is open, honest and respectful. Honest self-expression is not about getting things off your chest or dumping your feelings on to someone else. It's about owning your thoughts and feelings, deciding what is important and relevant to share and then communicating those thoughts and feelings as a grown-up adult. This is speaking your truth. It is about sharing your inner reality with another person, but doing so – and this is the key – with the simple intention of communicating and sharing what's true for you. It's not about control, getting results, power struggles, manipulating the other person or trying to get them to change. Put another way, you are not trying to get anything from the other person; you are just sharing your truth with them. That's the first half of the process; the second half, if appropriate and necessary, is to then listen to and receive the truth of what they have to say.

Of course this sounds daunting. And it is. But, like any skill, it gets easier the more you practise. When I explain the process of honest self-expression to my patients, many of them (just like I used to) are concerned at the prospect of 'opening up' to others. I completely understand why. Being vulnerable and speaking our truth brings up a lot of fear, and most of us, in the past, have not had positive experiences when speaking our truth. (If you want to learn more about this topic, I recommend the work of Marshall Rosenberg, the developer of nonviolent communication. See Recommended reading, page 291.)

EXERCISE: Honest self-expression

Practise with someone you trust and with whom you feel safe. Here are some suggestions to get you started:

- A good way to start the process is to share exactly how you are feeling in that moment. For example, 'I feel fearful and vulnerable talking to you about. . .'

- The key is to keep what you are sharing connected to and rooted in your feelings, i.e. resist the temptation to talk about the life situation or about someone else; just focus on what you feel about the life situation or feel in relationship to that person.

- Breathe deeply and allow yourself to feel what you are feeling as you speak. Avoid the temptation to rush – keep connected to what you are feeling.

- If you can, 'drop' beneath the feeling and identify the unmet need. There often is an unmet need there – what is it? Is it to be heard, appreciated, accepted or respected? Or is your need simply to share your perspective?

- Sharing your feelings and underlying needs might be enough. However, there are times, especially when you might be in conflict with someone, that you need to make a request that will fulfil the unmet need. Once shared this may or may not need to be negotiated.

- A successful outcome occurs when the communication process has been completed with respect and as a mature adult. You have communicated your feelings and needs and made a request to address the unmet needs and negotiated if necessary. You will know it's complete because you will feel a positive shift in your well-being and will feel at peace.

It's not easy, but it really does come with practice.

Tips

- When using honest self-expression with someone with whom you feel upset, one of the most important things is to become present. Use 4/7 breathing or one of the other emotional processing skills. You want to be in touch with your feelings but not overwhelmed by them.

- If you are in a conflict with someone, take a look at my suggestions for how to resolve conflict in Pillar Eight (see page 257). One of the keys to sharing your truth is to keep the focus on you by using 'I' statements, rather than 'you' statements. For example, 'I feel sad when you say that', rather than, 'You make me sad'. It is a revelation to realise the fact that no one causes you to feel a certain way; it is how you respond to what others do and say that makes you feel the way you do. So, you have choice in how you feel in any given moment.

- Avoid using the word 'feel' as part of a judgement: 'I feel that you are bad' or, 'I feel like you don't care'. When you notice yourself using phrases like this, just smile to yourself, and without judging yourself, rephrase what you have just said. So, rather than saying, 'I feel you are bad', say, 'When you speak to me like that, I feel sad, hurt and scared'.

A few questions to ask yourself

When using honest self-expression in everyday situations, it's important to be discerning both in terms of what you share, who you share it with, when you share and how much you share. Ask yourself the following questions before using honest self-expression. It will probably feel strange thinking about this initially, but with practice it should start to feel more natural.

Am I in a mature adult state in which I can express myself openly, honestly and with respect?   Before you speak, ask yourself how old you feel. If the answer is anything less than your chronological age, it suggests that you have emotionally regressed and the voice that is about to emerge from your mouth is from your immature adolescent self, not your adult self. If so, the most important thing to do is to 'grow yourself' back up, before speaking. You can do this by using any of the other processing tools (for example EmoTrance). I normally do 4/7 breathing (see page xxiii), focus on my heart and silently say the words 'I am the mature adult self'. Once you feel as though you are in your adult self, then that is the time to speak.

Is what I am about to say true?   It's important to ask this question. If what you're about to say isn't true, what can you say or do which would be more truthful and also respectful? This helps to break the automatic pattern that many people have of exaggerating, lying or saying things that simply aren't true.

Is what I am about to say appropriate to the situation?   This is where discernment comes in. I might be feeling upset about something my wife said to me prior to leaving for work and all set to talk about it when returning home; however, if she is in the middle of cooking dinner or about to get ready to go out for the evening, the moment probably isn't going to be right. Of course, sometimes the moment may never feel right, but the way to create the right moment is to say something along the lines of, 'There is something important I want to share with you. When will be the best time to speak?' You then negotiate an appropriate time.

Before you go any further I really encourage you to try at least one of the three emotional processing tools that I have just outlined. Just identify something you have strong emotions about and use your new tool. Most people find EmoTrance the easiest and then move onto Cradling and Honest Self-expression after a week or so. My final tip – get into the habit of using them whenever emotions come up. The more you do so, the easier you will find them. Eventually they will become second nature.

PILLAR TWO: Summary

- Emotions are just energy-in-motion.

- Emotions provide information about how well you are/are not meeting your emotional and physical needs.

- There is no such thing as a negative emotion, just emotions you negate.

- Most of us compulsively avoid, sedate or control certain emotions without realising that in so doing we limit our capacity for joy, aliveness and true intimacy with others.

- A healthy way to relate to emotions is to welcome them and then process (digest) them skilfully so that you receive their information, then act on it responsibly and maturely.

Pillar Three: Live a fulfilling and meaningful life

Is the life that you are currently living truly fulfilling and meaningful? Do you wake up in the morning with a real sense of how good it is to be alive? Are you dedicating your time and energy to the things that truly matter to you?

If your answer to any of these is, 'No', then this pillar is definitely for you. A fulfilling and meaningful life is as it sounds – full and meaningful. However, the fullness I am referring to has nothing to do with how busy your schedule is; it's to do with a deep-seated feeling of inner well-being, vitality and peace – the true happiness that comes from living life in a way that enables your potential, talents, strengths and gifts to shine through. It's about getting clear in your own mind what truly matters to you and then making sure that you live in alignment with those values.

People who consistently take action that satisfies their values and needs are healthier and happier and show greater levels of well-being after completing their goals, when compared with those who focus on goals that are not chosen on that basis.[16] It's about bringing all of yourself to life and engaging with it as fully as possible. Not doing this creates a type of pain that I call the pain of unfulfilled potential. It's a heaviness, an emptiness and restlessness deep within you that arises whenever you move off course from your values, strengths and unique gifts or whenever you act in a way that is not true to who you are and what you stand for.

It's so easy to get caught up in your own problems and your own thinking and lose sight of what is right about life and about yourself. But the purpose of life is to share our gifts, talents and strengths in a way that not only enhances our own well-being but that of others too. We are here to thrive and flourish as human beings – not in terms of material wealth, achievements and gain, but emotionally and spiritually.

Of course, you must address those issues that are causing mental distress and you must learn how to have a better relationship with yourself and with others. The key to true happiness, however, lies not in fixing problems, but in embracing a way of being and living that enables you to fulfil your potential. When this happens, you shift from fixing to awakening, and from being self-centred to being of service.

The foundations – healthy self-care and gratitude

To live in the world as an emotionally and psychologically mature adult you need solid foundations. Two of what I consider to be the most important foundations for creating a fulfilling and meaningful life are healthy self-care and gratitude. When these two are being actively nurtured each day, they provide the physical vitality, emotional balance and mental clarity for you to thrive and flourish. Let's start by looking at healthy self-care.

Healthy self-care

I define healthy self-care as the ongoing process of responding to the physical and emotional needs of your body and mind in a way that is balanced and moderate. Our physical needs (which are covered in Pillar Four) are for healthy food, water, physical activity, sleep, rest, relaxation, sunlight and a healthy environment. Our emotional needs, which not many people know about (and are discussed in this pillar), are for security, giving and receiving positive attention, connection with a wider community, an intimate close relationship with at least one other person, autonomy, status, competence, privacy, and meaning and purpose.

The intention of healthy self-care is not only to prevent illness and if necessary support your recovery from various health problems, but also to take care of your body–mind in a way that enables you to experience your fullest physical, emotional, psychological and social potential.

Why is healthy self-care so important?

Healthy self-care doesn't come naturally to most of us, and there are many reasons for this. We might, for example, not be aware of what our needs are (this is particularly the case if we are used to focusing on meeting the needs of others); we might have undiagnosed compulsions and addictions (which keep us out of the present moment); we might feel guilty about indulging ourselves by taking care of our needs; or, and this is very common, we are so busy, stressed and caught up in our thoughts that we simply don't have the mental space to be aware of what our body is asking of us. I also think that for many people it comes down to the fact that they don't really value their health and well-being.

CASE STUDY: LORRAINE

Lorraine, a thirty-seven-year-old mother of two, came to see me because she was experiencing repeated colds, indigestion and exhaustion. In addition to taking care of her children, she did the administration for her husband's company and was 'always available to her friends'. On most nights, she didn't get to sleep until 11 p.m. It wasn't hard to see that this kind, loving woman was simply overwhelmed by the way she was living her life. She had lost sight of who she was (beyond her roles as mother, wife and friend) and she no longer knew how to take care of her own needs because her energy and attention were on people and things outside of her. While perceived as a super-organised person, on the inside she was empty, alone, tired and unhappy.

It was pretty straightforward to diagnose her as suffering from stress-induced illness, co-dependency (we examine this in Pillar Eight), sleep deprivation, adrenal exhaustion, anxiety, hormone imbalance and a low-functioning immune system. However, the scale and depth of her challenges made it imperative that I did not overwhelm her even more with a long 'to-do' list.

My starting point with Lorraine, as it is for many of my patients, was to talk about the benefits of healthy self-care and the need for her to take responsibility for meeting her physical and emotional needs. We identified that her greatest physical need was for more sleep, and her greatest unmet emotional need was for an intimate, close relationship with at least one other person. Lorraine agreed that for the next two weeks she would make some positive changes in her life. She announced to her friends that she was unavailable after 8 p.m. and ensured that she was asleep by 10 p.m. each night. Her husband agreed to get up every other night if any of the kids woke up. On the emotional need front, she opened up to a close friend about what had been going on for her, and they have since been speaking every other day. For the first time, and within just two weeks, Lorraine felt more rested, supported and happy.

The benefits of embracing healthy self-care

If Lorraine's case hasn't quite convinced you of the value of healthy self-care, consider the findings of a recent Department of Health report. It found that people who embrace and prioritise healthy self-care experience: [17]

- An improved ability to withstand and cope with stress

- A more positive outlook on life

- Better health and significantly improved quality of life

- Increased life expectancy

- Reduction in symptoms, such as insomnia, pain, depression and asthma

- Improved ability to make more informed decisions about health and well-being

- Increased self-esteem and sense of mastery

- A reduction in shame and feelings of estrangement

- Reduced psychosomatic symptoms

- Improved relationships

In addition, they reduce demand on health services and are less likely to require medications. Convinced? I hope so. Let's start by looking at our emotional needs and how we can go about meeting them.

Meet your emotional needs

To experience emotional health and reach emotional maturity each of us needs to meet certain emotional needs. Leaving them unmet is a major contributor to emotional and mental distress. My approach to emotional needs is based on the pioneering work of an organisation called the Human Givens Institute[18] (see Resources, page 276). The term 'Human Givens' refers to four related ideas:

1. Our capacity to experience mental health, personal growth and optimum functioning is dependent upon our ability to satisfy nine genetically programmed emotional needs in an ongoing and balanced way. These needs are universal in that they apply to all people, regardless of culture or gender.

2. We are instinctively trying to fulfil these needs using specific resources that we are born with.

3. Our emotions are what drive us to take action so that we can get these needs met.

4. If we are unable to meet our emotional needs and/or apply our resources adequately this will inevitably lead to distress (anger, fear, anxiety and stress) and mental ill-health.

What are our emotional needs?

As I pointed out at the start of this pillar, our nine emotional needs are: security, giving and receiving positive attention, connection with a wider community, an intimate close relationship with at least one other person, autonomy, status, competence, privacy, and meaning and purpose. Let's look at each of these.

1. Security

This includes the security of living in a safe environment and neighbourhood and the safety of knowing that you are physically and emotionally safe in the presence of the people that surround you (both at home and your place of work). Security also includes feeling secure in your work, job and relationship. Feeling safe and knowing how to deal effectively with fear provides us with the necessary environment in which to develop and grow our potential.

2. Giving and receiving positive attention

You just have to watch a child to witness how powerful this need is. But it isn't confined to children – adults also need to give and receive positive attention. Much of what we do and say and how we dress, interact and project ourselves is influenced by our need for quality, sincere attention. Many of my patients are good at giving, but less so at receiving and digesting the energy of positive attention. This is often rooted in low self-esteem and co- and counter-dependency (see Pillar Eight, page 245).

3. Connection with a wider community

We are intrinsically social creatures and need to feel that we are part of something beyond our immediate family group. Having a wider social network and enjoying the company of people with similar or common interests is a key need if you are to create total health. Having a network of friends and participating in groups or community-related projects are well known to protect against depression.

4. An intimate close relationship with at least one other person

Intimacy means having meaningful emotional contact with another person. While the depth of the interaction will naturally vary, in respect of emotional growth and healing the most benefit is derived from being able to share the truth of yourself – the good, the bad and the ugly – with them. When this is received with understanding and acceptance, the process of healing is supported. This kind of relationship could include your partner, a friend, therapist and/or spiritual/religious teacher.

5. Autonomy

A person who feels that they have some degree of control in respect of their life situation (work, finances and relationships) is able to withstand stress and life's challenges much more effectively than someone who has little or no control. Taking responsibility for your health and emotional well-being demonstrates that you are already increasing your autonomy.

6. Status

In any given social situation, we each need to feel that we have our place and purpose – a sense that we are being recognised and respected for who we are. This needs to include our place within the home and at work. Status is something we give to ourselves and receive from others.

7. Competence

Self-esteem – the estimation of yourself – is intimately tied up with feeling competent and having a sense of accomplishment in what you do. This can apply in many aspects of your life, including relationships, lovemaking, work, recreation and sports, and comes about by taking action that is in alignment with your gifts, strengths and values.

8. Privacy

This is not so much about removing yourself from contact with others, but knowing that you can control the amount of contact you have with others, and use your private time to reflect on and consolidate your experiences. It's also about balance and moderation, i.e. not isolating yourself from others but taking time out regularly to rejuvenate.

9. Meaning and purpose

Our minds are constantly trying to attach meaning to what we do and what we experience. When something has meaning, it takes on importance and adds depth and flavour to life, for better or for worse. Tied in with meaning is purpose – the feelings of determination and drive that come from having a vision and belief in what you are doing. Taking actions that are aligned with your values, growing and evolving as a human being and being stretched and engaged with the world are some of the keys to creating positive meaning and purpose.

In addition to the nine emotional needs, nature has also endowed us with the specific resources to meet them. These include:

- Curiosity – the ability to develop learn and acquire new knowledge and insight

- The ability to build rapport, empathise and connect with others

- Imagination, which provides the ability to solve problems, plan the future, instruct the subconscious mind and alter memories that might have adverse effects

- A conscious, rational mind that can analyse, make plans and control emotions

- The ability to 'know' – understand the world unconsciously through metaphorical pattern-matching

- An observing self – a part of us that can step back from and observe our emotions and thoughts

- Dreaming – nature's way of discharging stress (see page 52)

Using these resources to meet your emotional needs in a healthy and balanced way is one of the most important keys to emotional and mental health. A failure to meet emotional needs leads to emotional and psychological distress – whether you are aware of it or not. Left unresolved, this accumulated distress often deteriorates into anxiety, addictions, depression and, in the predisposed, psychosis. The key, therefore, is to identify which of your emotional needs is not being met. I ask all my patients to fill in the questionnaire below and I invite you to do the same.

QUESTIONNAIRE: Are your emotional needs being met?

Read through each question slowly and rate how well the various emotional needs are being met in your life now. For each one, give yourself a score of between 1 and 7 (where 1 = emotional need completely unmet and unfulfilled and 7 = emotional need completely met and fulfilled). Leave out any questions that are not applicable.

Note: watch out for the tendency to rush this exercise or to score yourself too highly. Once you have a score in mind, ask yourself, 'Does this feel accurate?' If it does, write it down; if not, reassess and score again.

- Do you feel secure in all major areas of your life? ☐

- Do you feel that you are receiving enough positive attention? ☐

- Do you think you give other people enough positive attention? ☐

- Do you feel that you have a choice as to how you live your life? ☐

- Do you feel connected to some part of the wider community? ☐

- Do you take time for reflection when you need and want to? ☐

- Do you have at least one intimate relationship in which you are totally accepted for who you are? ☐

- Do you feel emotionally connected to your partner? ☐

- Do you feel emotionally connected to your close friends? ☐

- Do you feel emotionally connected to your family? ☐

- Do you feel competent in your main occupation? ☐

- Do you have a sense of accomplishment in what you do on most days? ☐

- Are you respected and acknowledged by your friends? ☐

- Are you respected and acknowledged by your work peers? ☐

- Are you respected and acknowledged by your family? ☐

- Are you respected and acknowledged by your partner? ☐

- Overall, do you feel that your life is meaningful and fulfilling? ☐

Having completed the questionnaire, go through it again and consider whether the scores you have given yourself are an accurate reflection of reality. Generally, the lower the score for a particular emotional need, the greater the need for action. My experience has shown that a score of five or less represents a barrier to well-being, and that three or less indicates an unmet need that is almost certainly contributing to stress and/or a mental health problem. Write down your three lowest-scoring emotional needs in a notebook or journal.

How to meet your emotional needs

Now that you know what your unmet emotional needs are, it's time to start taking practical action to meet them. If you are experiencing distress and/or a mental-health problem you may need a friend or even a human potential coach to support you (see Resources, page 275). However, it is possible to make very positive changes by yourself.

I'll now guide you through the same process that I use with my patients. I have provided a template below using the example of the need for giving and receiving positive attention. Write the questions in your notebook, replacing the example given in italics with the unmet need that you want to work on. You will then need to write your responses to each of the questions. Start with the unmet emotional need that is troubling you the most.

The emotional need-fulfilment process

- What does *giving and receiving positive attention* mean to me? If my need for *giving and receiving positive attention* was fulfilled, what would be different and positive about my life right now? (Close your eyes and imagine that this is true for you – what would you see, hear, feel, notice? Give yourself plenty of time to do this.)

- I wonder how I can *give and allow myself to receive more positive attention*? What underlying beliefs are contributing to my issues around *attention*? How can I transform them? (See Pillar One – 'Transform any self-limiting beliefs', page 30.)

- What practical steps can I take today in order to increase my ability to *give and receive positive attention*?

- Who can I ask for support and help in relationship to this issue?

Here are some suggestions for where to look in this book for support in addressing your unmet emotional needs:

- **For security** – see Pillar Two, 'Become skilful in emotional processing', page 51 (particularly fear); all of Pillar Seven; and Pillar Eight, 'Identify the presence of co-dependency/counter-dependency behaviours' (page 245) and 'Develop and maintain healthy boundaries' (page 251).

- **For giving and receiving positive attention** – see all of Pillar Seven and Pillar Eight, 'Practise empathy' (page 237) and 'Practise the four As of healthy relationships' (page 241).

- **Connection with a wider community** – consider doing voluntary work, attending local events, getting involved with your local church, attending an evening class, joining a local special-interest group or making an effort to get to know your neighbours.

- **An intimate close relationship with at least one other person** – see all of Pillars Seven and Eight.

- **Autonomy** – see How to Make This Book Work For You (the section on committed action, page xxi); the rest of this pillar, especially the section on values, page 77), Pillar Six, 'Psychological stress' (page 182); and Pillar Eight, 'Identify the presence of co-dependency/counter-dependency behaviours' (page 245) and 'Develop and maintain healthy boundaries' (page 251).

- **Status** – see all of Pillars Seven and Eight.

- **Competence** – see the rest of this pillar, especially the sections on values, gifts and strengths, pages 76 and 77) and Pillar Seven (all of it).

- **Privacy** – build time into your day in which you can be both alone and able to reflect on your experiences (see the section on rest and relaxation in Pillar Four, page 117).

- **Meaning and purpose** – see the rest of this pillar, especially the section on values, page 77) and Pillar Seven (all of it). Meaning and purpose also come from spiritual and religious practices, having a life-enhancing philosophy of life and developing new skills. How can you develop any one of these?

CASE STUDY: CHRIS

Chris did the emotional needs questionnaire on page 68 and scored low in security, competence and wider community. Here are the solutions he came up with (with the help of a good friend):

- Security – put additional bolts on the door, install a burglar alarm or move house
- Competence – ask boss for more training, ask boss to be moved to the human resources team (I have a lot of HR experience), find a new job, take an online course or evening course in business management
- Wider community – take evening classes, volunteer at local woodland trust, go to meditation classes in local village hall, join rotary club

Chris began putting some of these into action straight away. Despite his fears and reservations about talking to his boss, his boss agreed to move him into HR, and within a month he was doing work that he felt competent in. He felt much safer having fitted the bolts and burglar alarm; he also subsequently started a Neighbourhood Watch scheme, much to the delight of some of the local residents, and he took up voluntary work and regular meditation classes. Within four weeks, his depression and anxiety had lifted and he felt 'more empowered and at peace' than he had ever been. All because he started meeting his emotional needs.

Embrace gratitude

One of the most effective (and often quickest) ways to shift the way you feel, lift your mood and enhance your well-being is to practise gratitude. Robert Emmons, the world's leading gratitude researcher, describes gratitude as the 'felt sense of wonder, thankfulness and appreciation for life'. Along with healthy self-care, gratitude provides the foundations upon which a fulfilling and meaningful life is built.

One of the many fascinating discoveries to emerge from the field of positive psychology – the study of how human beings flourish – is that the regular and deliberate practice of gratitude can bring about significant relief from stress and considerable improvements in happiness, motivation, optimism, energy levels, sleep and quality of life. It is also a powerful antidote to 'negative emotions' and depression, as well as the foundation upon which a fulfilling life is created. In my own work I have found that it is as important to practise cultivating positive emotional states, such as gratitude, as it is to deal with anger, grief and mental illness.

Here are two suggestions for increasing the level of gratitude in your life. I suggest you do both for a week and then stick with the one you enjoy most.

EXERCISE: The gratitude ritual

The following is a five-minute ritual that I highly recommend you do every morning for seven days. It's a highly effective way to shift yourself into a deep sense of gratitude.

Read through the steps below once, then try them out yourself. Although this can be done in your head, for best results you should write step three out on a piece of paper or, preferably, in a journal.

1. Today is a new day. The past is past and today I choose to take actions that will support me waking up and growing up and move me more fully into my potential as a human being.

2. Today I open myself to guidance, to true happiness and new ways of bringing joy to myself and others.

3. Today I am truly grateful for . . . [write down at least three things].

4. Now, taking into account your gifts, strengths and values (which you will discover in the remainder of this pillar), close your eyes and create a mental picture of what a fulfilling and meaningful life would look like for you. Experience yourself living this life as though it is happening now. Take time to see what it looks like. How would you be spending your time? Who would you be surrounded by? How would you be as a person? Don't worry about seeing it clearly; getting a sense of it will be enough.

5. Keeping your eyes closed, turn your attention to what you are now feeling. Allow yourself to welcome it and feel it fully for ten seconds or so.

6. Eyes still closed, imagine that this new life was really happening and focus on the gratitude that you have because this is so. Allow those feelings of gratitude to arise in you and, as they do, feel them fully. Enjoy the feelings you are now experiencing. When you are ready, move on with your day.

EXERCISE: Keep a gratitude journal

Write in a journal some of the things you have to be grateful for. This can be anything from the beauty of the sky outside to the joy of your children – whatever works for you. Some people really enjoy doing this every day, others once a week – you will find out what suits you.

I get my patients to start by writing down two things for which they are grateful and two things that they appreciate about themselves. For example:

Today, I am grateful for:

1. The aliveness that I'm feeling in my body, as it provides me with the inspiration and energy to do my work

2. The fingers I have, as they allow me to write this message

Today I appreciate:

1. The loving respect with which I greeted my daughter this morning

2. The friendly manner with which I spoke to Susan on the phone

Once you have written your list, allow yourself to feel the gratitude in your body for at least thirty seconds. One of the defining features and experiences of someone who is living in alignment with their true self, is the gratefulness that they have for simply being alive. A good barometer of how in touch you are with your true self is the amount of gratitude that you are aware of in each moment. Take a moment to get in touch with it whenever you can.

Identify your life purpose and gifts

Imagine that within you is a gift that when expressed will bring you and the people around you a great deal of joy. And imagine that one of the master keys to true happiness and inner fulfilment was to discover and start using that gift. You'd be pretty keen to find out what it is, wouldn't you?

The idea of us each having a gift was something that I discovered when I took an honest look at what brought me and others the most joy in life. I noticed that there were certain moments in which I experienced a deep sense of fulfilment and inner peace and that those moments happened repeatedly whenever I was in a specific situation and able to allow certain qualities to emerge.

This led me to develop the exercise below, which I have since used with my patients to help them discover their 'outer life purpose' (what will bring them and others the greatest fulfilment and joy) and their 'inner gift' (the qualities from within that are waiting to be expressed through their outer life purpose). The process I use also helps to identify the necessary conditions that allow this to happen. As people use this discovery process and start to focus on using their gifts whenever they can, their fulfilment and happiness levels increase substantially. It's not a panacea, but it is an important part of the jigsaw for transforming your life.

EXERCISE: Discover your life purpose and gifts

1. **What is your life purpose?** Think about what you love to do or would love to do that would bring you a deep sense of fulfilment, as well as making a positive contribution to the well-being of others and/or the planet. If you had no money worries whatsoever, what would you be doing simply because of the joy it brings to you and others? My response to this is: 'To create a life equal to my potential and to help others do the same.' Write your own in a journal or notebook.

2. **What is your inner gift?** When you are doing what you love, what are the exact qualities that you are allowing to emerge? This takes you much deeper and reveals your inner gift. My response to this is: 'I am allowing clarity, wisdom, insight and kindness to emerge through me.' Write your own in a journal or notebook.

3. **What liberates your gifts?** How do you need to be in order to experience your inner and outer gifts? What needs to happen in

order for you to experience them? My response to this is: 'By being present, relaxed and open.' Write your own.

So, to summarise, using my own responses, I discovered that:

- My outer life purpose is to create a life equal to my potential and to help others do the same.

- My inner gifts waiting to emerge through me are clarity, wisdom, insight and kindness.

- I will experience and bring forth my gifts by being present, relaxed, open and trusting.

You might struggle at first to identify your gifts; I did initially. The key is not to rush the process, but to keep playing with your answers until they feel right. You will know when you have discovered the right answer because you will feel a warmth and sense of expansion in your body. You will just know that you have hit the bull's eye. Another good way to do this work is to do it with a friend or partner. Get them to ask the questions and to write down your answers. Alternatively, give it a break for a few days and then come back to it. Being as relaxed as you can be while doing it makes it much easier for your truth to reveal itself to you.

Once you've discovered your outer life purpose, your inner gift and how to access it, what next? Two things: 1) you allocate more of your time, energy and life to situations in which you are expressing your gift and 2) you start developing the skills that enable your gifts to emerge – in my case the skill was present-moment awareness.

IDENTIFY YOUR STRENGTHS

One of the keys to happiness and fulfilment is to live life in a way that maximises your strengths and talents and minimises the impact of your weaknesses. A strength is something that you are good at, comes naturally to you and energises you. A weakness is something that you find hard to do and when you do, it drains you. We all have strengths and weaknesses – that's part of being human. To help you identify your strengths I recommend using one of the following strengths assessment tools. The first one is called the VIA Strengths questionnaire and it's free. You can find it at www.viastrengths.org. The other one is Realise 2.0, which will help identify your strengths and your weaknesses. You can access it at www.cappeu.com for a small charge. Having identified what they are the next step is to start designing your day and your life in a way that harnesses your strengths, as well as your gifts and values.

Discover your values

What do you truly value? What is of utmost importance to you in your life? If you took a look at how you spend your life right now what would you discover about what is important to you? Getting clarity around the answers to these questions, discovering your values and then living in alignment with your highest ones is absolutely at the heart of creating a fulfilling and meaningful life.

What are values?

Values embody what is most important to you, they define what really, truly matters to you at the deepest possible level. It's important to distinguish values from goals. Values provide the direction, goals the destination. Values exist in the here and now – you can always honour a value, whereas goals exist in the future. For example, a value of mine is honesty. In any given moment I can honour that value. A goal that is aligned with that value might be to phone my best friend regularly and share with him how I'm feeling.

However, the problem for nearly all of us is that:

- So few of us are aware of what our values are

- We haven't assessed whether the values we have and the priorities we assign to them are bringing us the quality of life we desire

- We're unaware of the self-imposed rules around our values

- We have unprocessed fears that sabotage our ability to live in alignment with our values

So, values are not actions, things, possessions or destinations (goals), but ongoing actions, i.e. you can be doing and honouring them on an ongoing basis right here, right now. Here is a list of some common values: honesty, integrity, intimacy, authenticity, acceptance, adventure, connection, contribution, fairness, kindness, love, humility, gratitude, freedom, fitness, creativity, courage, cooperation, compassion, caring, spirituality, beauty, excellence, assertiveness, mindfulness, trust and challenge.

The value of values

Why is working with your values important? In a nutshell, when you honour them they will bring you fulfilment. What's more, values heavily influence your life choices and decisions, so if you sense that your life isn't working for you, choosing new values or reprioritising existing values may help you to change your life direction considerably. Also, the human brain appears to be hard-wired for happiness via goal-seeking behaviour. So, setting goals that are aligned with your values and moving towards them will trigger the release of positive emotions, in order to motivate you and reinforce behaviours that support you in maturing as a human being.[19] This explains why so many therapists and psychologists are now encouraging their patients to take values-directed actions that are intrinsically rewarding, in addition to training their capacity to hold their attention (mindfulness), so that they can consciously choose what to focus on and engage with.

EXERCISE: Identify your values

The following questions will help you identify your existing values. Record your answers in a journal or on a piece of paper.

- If you had as much money as you needed and were living a comfortable lifestyle, what would the most fulfilling life possible look like for you? Spend some time reflecting on this and/or discussing it with a friend/partner. What values would you be honouring by living this life? Write them down.

- If you had the time or money, what would you most want to study, practise, master or research? What would you want to become an expert in? What values would you be honouring by living this life? Write them down.

- Make a list of things beyond food, shelter and clothing that you must have in order to be fulfilled and happy. For each of these things, what values are being honoured? Write them down.

- What causes are you willing to dedicate your life to? What values would you be honouring by living this life? Write them down.

- Identify a series of events that made you feel particularly angry or upset. Choose one of these and think about it for a moment. Now identify what value was not being expressed in that moment. Write it down. For example, Rita, a patient of mine, told me that she gets angry when her husband lies or exaggerates (she has a sixth sense that tells her when he is doing this), and from this she was able to see that the value of being honest wasn't being respected. Honesty was therefore one of her values.

- Identify a peak moment in time, in which you were completely at peace and in the moment. What values were being honoured in that moment? Write them down. Rita described the feeling of empowerment and peace that she experienced when she was pre-senting to her business colleagues. The main value that was hon-oured in that moment was the feeling of connection.

Once you have a list of your values, the next step is to identify your top ten, prioritised in terms of how important they are to you, then to score out of ten the degree to which they are being honoured in your life right now (where 1 = not being honoured at all and 10 = completely honoured; anything scoring less than 7 points indicates an area that needs to be addressed). Often, values can go together – for example, honesty/integrity or health/vitality (but if you do this, make sure they are compatible; freedom and security, for example are not) and lead with the one that is of greatest value to you. This takes a lot of time and reflection – you might want to write them in pencil first so that you can rearrange them as you wish. Working with a life coach can also help with this (see Resources, page 275).

Here are Rita's top ten values and their scores:

Value	Score
1. Spirituality	7
2. Compassion	4
3. Honesty/integrity	3
4. Creative self-expression	3
5. Authenticity	6
6. Health/fitness	5
7. Service	8
8. Love/connection	3
9. Fun/laughter	7
10. Freedom/independence	5

It's not hard to see why Rita wasn't experiencing fulfilment in her life with so few of her values being honoured. Now make your own list in a journal or notebook.

Recognising the barriers to values-based living

Having identified your current values, the next step is to identify clearly those that will and those that will not help you to live to your highest potential and move you towards a fulfilling life. (You will benefit immensely from increasing the priority of certain values – maybe new ones – and decreasing the priority of old ones.) Remember, values shape your life and life direction, so this exercise has the potential to make a significant difference to the quality of your life.

For each of the values that you identified in the exercise, ask yourself, 'Is this a value that will support me in waking up and growing up and help me live the most fulfilling life possible?' If so, write it down; if not, write down those values that *will* help you achieve this – and start to prioritise them. Be prepared, as before, to swap them round and change your mind quite a few times. That's just part of the process.

Your rules for living in alignment with your values

So, you've identified what truly is important to you – your values – and all you have to do now is live in alignment with this in order to experience happiness and fulfilment. Unfortunately, however, it's not that simple because we also have rules about how to fulfil our values, and many of us have fears that hold us back from honouring them.

You can elicit your rules by taking each of your values in turn and asking the question: 'What needs to happen in order for that value to be fulfilled?' Here is what one workshop participant, Laura, wrote:

- **Health – improving my physical health** I need to be slim, have no skin blemishes, have high energy levels and no health problems.

- **Connections – developing and deepening connections** I need people to be kind to me and to respect me; I need to feel special and appreciated; I need to feel safe with the person I am with.

- **Autonomy – freedom to be me** I need to be able to do what I want when I want; I need people to not control me.

- **Having fun** I need the people who come out with me in the evenings to be relaxed and having fun; I need to have new and exciting experiences when I'm with my friends.

The type of rules that Laura shared are not that uncommon, but there is a major problem. Laura's rules require things to happen that are out of her control. Take 'I need people to be kind to me and to respect me', for example: unfortunately, it's never going to happen, because she can't control other people's behaviour and feelings. For this reason, Laura will feel unloved most of the time (and she confirmed that this is true). So what's the solution? The key to fulfilling your rules is to rewrite them as positively stated ones over which you have complete control (and the more rules per value, the better). Here are the new rules that Laura came up with:

- **Health – improving my physical health** I will feel healthy/vital any time I eat healthy food, drink water, get rest and relaxation, meet my physical and emotional needs, exercise and spend time in nature.

- **Connections – developing and deepening connections** I will allow myself to feel love when I respect myself and treat myself with kindness and compassion, when I am kind and compassionate towards others, when I respectfully speak my truth and when I help or inspire others.

- **Autonomy – freedom to be me** I will allow myself to feel freedom when I speak my truth, set clear boundaries and take responsibility for my feelings, words and actions.

- **Having fun** I will allow myself to experience fun by enjoying and making the most of any situation.

What a difference! Laura's new rules gave her – crucially – control over each action. She moved from disempowerment to empowerment in just a few minutes.

What are your value-attached fears and feelings?

You are getting closer to discovering how to live a values-driven life, but there is one more important piece of work to do.

When I compiled my own values list I placed honesty, integrity and sincerity at number one. I did so because when I am able to be honest and act with integrity and sincerity, I notice that all of my other values are much more likely to be fulfilled as a result. However, despite choosing things that were achievable and within my personal control as my highest values and rules, there were – and still are – occasions when I didn't speak my truth. This is because I have fears that are pulling me away from and sabotaging my ability to fulfil my values. I have, in the past, experienced pain when speaking my truth and pleasure (relief/comfort/safety) by not doing so (usually by withholding or saying what I thought the other person *wanted* to hear). And, because my brain – like everyone's – is programmed to avoid pain and seek pleasure, any time I want to speak my truth, past memories of pain would prevent me. The result is a conflict between values I hold dear – honesty, integrity and sincerity – and the fear of rejection or humiliation.

I started to overcome this by identifying the fear (or fears) that existed in relationship to my values – so-called value-attached fears.

To do this, simply select each value in turn, and imagine living and experiencing them. Write down exactly what that value means to you, in the form of a value statement (see below). Next, ask yourself the following question: 'What fears come up for me when I imagine living a life that embraces . . .' (honesty, integrity and sincerity, for example). You then write down your fears next to your values or value statement. Here are just some of the values and fears that I had.

Values statement	Fears
To live with honesty, integrity and sincerity	That others will reject me and will be upset by what I say/how I am
To realise my gifts and potential	That I won't be able to stay committed and focused; that I will be moved in a direction my ego doesn't want to go.
To deepen my connection to spirit	That I will lose interest in worldly things, including family and work; I won't have control over my life
To be a loving, caring, supportive partner	That I will be emotionally hurt, that I will be smothered
To be a loving, caring, supportive father	That I will not know how to be with my children; that I won't be good enough
To have a healthy and vital body and mind	That I won't be able to stay committed and focused; that I will lose motivation. That it will be hard work to keep it up and it will consume a lot of time/energy
To be broaden and deepen my understanding of the process of health	That I will be regarded as 'weak' or 'wet'; that I will be taken advantage of

This is an example of some of my value-attached fears. You should identify the fears that are attached to all your values. The next step is to process them so that they are no longer strong enough to prevent you from consistently meeting your values. There are many different ways in which to do that; here are just a couple:

- Acknowledge your fears and share/talk about them with a friend.

- Process your fears/feelings fully (Cradling and EmoTrance are particularly useful, see Pillar Two, pages 53 and 55).

Live in alignment with your highest values

Having identified your life purpose, gifts and highest values, and started to address any underlying fears and feelings connected to them, the next and most important step is to take daily action to ensure that you are living in alignment with your values. This will liberate the vitality and fulfilment within you.

Try to focus on your top three or four values and, at the beginning of and throughout the day, ask yourself whether you are acting in alignment with them. For example, if your top four values were honesty, integrity, health and connection, you would ask yourself the following:

- How can I share honestly when speaking with people today?

- How can I act with integrity today?

- How can I be healthy and vital in body, mind and spirit today?

- How can I feel more connected and loving towards myself and others today?

Shall I, shan't I?

In addition to asking yourself such questions at the start of every day (and they do need to be asked every day), there will be plenty of times when you have a decision to make about some direction in your life. A good way to work out whether this decision will positively impact your life and bring you more fulfilment is to see how it will impact on your values. If, for example, I am offered an opportunity that will increase the fulfilment of my contribution values, but in doing so it reduces higher values, such as connection and intimacy, it's likely that overall it won't be the right decision for me. If, however, it increases my higher-ranked values it probably is.

Setting value-based goals

Some people love to set goals, as it provides them with a focus and limits distraction. I am all for this as long as the goals are realistic, flexible, authentic (they come from you and not anyone else), positively motivated and rooted in values and emotional needs. Here is a process that I use to help my workshop participants set goals for themselves:

EXERCISE: Set your value-based goals

1. Bearing in mind your life purpose, gifts and highest values, decide on the specific goal or outcome that you would like.

2. How desirable and challenging is this goal (1 = not challenging, 10 = extremely challenging)? It should score at least five.

3. Think about your goal, breathe deeply and turn your attention to your body – do you feel conflict or harmony? Signs of conflict include feeling contracted, uneasy or uncomfortable; confusion; feeling heavy, sleepy and/or tired; doubt; boredom. Signs of harmony include feeling expanded, light and at peace; clarity and alertness; feeling uplifted, energised and/or content; knowing; enthusiasm and motivation.

4. If you feel conflict, which aspect of your goal is causing this? Look at each part of your goal in turn and tune into the feedback from your body. Alternatively, ask yourself: 'Am I choosing this goal because of some underlying fear, belief or worry?' If so, what is that? Create a goal around it. For example, the goal of becoming a millionaire in order to feel successful could become the goal of cultivating self-acceptance, out of which might come financial success.

5. Modify and rewrite your goal until you feel signs of harmony. Write down your new goal.

6. Now close your eyes, breathe deeply and create a movie of what your life would look like and how you would feel once this goal was accomplished. Give yourself plenty of time for this. It's important that you associate with the image of yourself – in other words, you should experience yourself as the person in the movie. If it helps, use the following questions to inspire you:

   • What do you see that shows you have solved the problem or achieved the goal?

   • What are other people doing or saying that tells you that you have succeeded?

   • What does it feel like?

   • When do you realistically want to be in the position that you see in your mind's eye?

   • How will you know that you have achieved your goal?

   • Is there a measure you can use?

   • How much control or influence do you have with regard to this goal?

7. Now turn your attention to the past. Try to identify a moment or experience from the past when you successfully completed a goal. Relive it and allow yourself to become energised by it. Once you feel that energy running through you, let go of the old memory and animate your new movie with this energy. Infuse it with life and make it as real as possible.

8. Repeat this process three more times. You will know when it's complete because when you think of your goal you will see and feel it as an energised reality. It will feel real.

9. If you get disorientated, confused or become unsure of what you are doing, just open your eyes, take a deep breath or have a glass of water and start again.

10. Once you have completed this process, the real key to achieving the goal is to reconnect with it at the start of every day. This

tuning-in process is important, particularly when it is preceded by a few moments of giving thanks and appreciation for what you have in your life.

Creating goals from a place of fulfilment, rather than poverty, appears to be another critical factor in helping to achieve them.

Be open to the fact that as life circumstances change, and as you continue to grow and evolve, your goals will usually change and evolve also. It's a good habit to regularly review them, as with values, to ensure that they still reflect what is true for you. Once a month is about right for most people.

PILLAR THREE: Summary

- The foundations of a fulfilling and meaningful life are gratitude and healthy self-care.

- Fulfilment and meaning come from meeting your emotional needs and taking actions that are aligned with your values, strengths and gifts.

- The purpose of life is to share our gifts, talents and strengths in a way that enhances and supports the well-being and evolution of ourselves and others.

Part Two

Overcoming common barriers to emotional health

Pillar Four: Meet your physical needs

Your emotional health and happiness are as much to do with the health and function of your brain and body, as they are with your mind. I am constantly amazed at how, time and time again, making simple adjustments to my patients' diets – say, reducing sugar and caffeine and removing foods to which they are intolerant – can bring about such positive changes in mood and well-being, and so quickly. What's more, by identifying and correcting hormone and neurotransmitter imbalances, checking for toxicity and correcting allergies, the positive changes that occur can be more profound and lasting than those that focus just on using emotion- or mind-based approaches.

It's highly unfortunate that the majority of doctors, psychiatrists, psychotherapists, counsellors and social workers – the five groups of people who work with people's emotional health problems – have not taken on board the food–mood link. Their ignorance of (or unwillingness to entertain) the link leads to sub-optimum care in most cases and months of unnecessary psychological treatments in many.

Take the case of a patient of mine called Sarah, which clearly demonstrates the importance of addressing dietary changes either before or in parallel with the necessary emotional, psychological or spiritual work.

CASE STUDY: SARAH

Sarah came to me because of ongoing anxiety and depression. While she described her temperament as 'nervy' and prone to worry, her symptoms of low mood, restlessness, insomnia and unpleasant thoughts had deteriorated over the previous few years. Her GP had placed her on medication and referred her for cognitive behavioural therapy (CBT). Although she felt the medication helped a little and the CBT was useful for dealing with her negative thinking, her quality of life was still poor and her symptoms still 'bad'.

What struck me about Sarah was how overwhelmed and exhausted she looked. After asking a number of questions about her diet and arranging some testing, it turned out that a significant contributor to her symptoms was (and had probably always been) the fact that she was sensitive to sugar. She craved sugar and ate up to six bars of chocolate a day; in her own words, she was 'unable to live without it'. What's more, her diet didn't stabilise her blood sugar or provide her with optimum levels of nutrients (both of which are essential for the best possible mental health). Plus, testing showed that she was deficient in omega-3 essential fatty acids, as well as some of the B vitamins and some minerals, such as zinc and magnesium.

While I always work in a holistic way with my patients, i.e. with mind and body in parallel, I decided with Sarah to start with a nutritional approach in order to assess the impact it would have. My instructions to her were to avoid sugar and all the foods she was intolerant to (tests revealed dairy and gluten intolerance) and to follow the principles of the nutrition programme that I am going share with you. When I assessed her in clinic just two weeks after making these changes, she reported a dramatic improvement in her mood, energy and health. It turns out that what she had been eating was a significant contributor to her symptoms of depression and anxiety and that addressing this issue first, she was much better placed – with a clearer mind and higher levels of energy and motivation – to address the other areas that needed to be looked at (including processing past trauma and learning new emotional-management skills).

Within six months, Sarah's depression and anxiety had disappeared and she was living a much healthier and more fulfilling life.

Healing the mind through the body

The body is a portal into the mind. If you think of the body as being the externalised, outermost expression of the mind, and each of them constantly exchanging information with the other, it's not that difficult to grasp the idea that the mind can be accessed and influenced through the body.

In fact, many emotionally focused therapies use the body-into-the-mind link in order to bring about emotional healing, personal growth and improved mental health. To discuss this fascinating area in any detail goes beyond the scope of this book; in essence though, many body-based approaches work to correct the flow of information around the body by correcting structural imbalances within it, freeing up the body's own healing mechanisms, allowing them to take over. Such approaches, including cranio-sacral therapy, rolfing, t'ai chi, yoga, massage, the Alexander technique, Pilates and acupuncture, while appearing to be working just on the physical body, are also working directly with the emotional body. They can influence your mood and health because of their ability to work at the more subtle level of energy and vibration. Many people use these to help manage stress and to support emotional healing; most of them will work nicely alongside my suggestions.

Transform your mood by meeting your physical needs

Your body and brain have an immense capacity for healing and improving your health and well-being, as long as certain physical needs are met. These include the need for a nutrient-rich diet; supplements (unfortunately diet alone doesn't provide enough nutrients); rest; relaxation; sleep; physical activity; sunlight; a healthy environment; and minimal exposure to smoking, excessive amounts of sugar, caffeine and alcohol.

Many health and emotional problems will often improve or even resolve just by meeting these needs. When provided in balance and moderation they enable the body–mind to do what it does best – that is to heal and restore balance.

Optimise your nutrition

Given that your brain, nervous system, neurotransmitters (chemicals that communicate mood) and body are built with and replenished by the nutrients that you take into your body, the strong connection between food and mood shouldn't come as a surprise. For example, a survey reported in 2002 by the Food and Mood project found that 88 per cent of those studied reported that changing their diet improved their mental health significantly. Twenty-six per cent said they saw substantial improvements in mood swings, 26 per cent in panic attacks and anxiety and 24 per cent in depression. Participants said that cutting down on food 'stressors' (foods like sugar, caffeine, alcohol and chocolate) and increasing the amount of 'supporters' (including water, vegetables, fruit and oil-rich fish) helped to improve their mood.[20]

Healthy eating is essential for good mental health and for your happiness, yet while most people know this to some degree, few actually make the necessary permanent modifications and improvements.

In this section, I'm going to show you how to get your diet right. It may seem quite scientific in places, but don't be put off – it's not as technical as it may at first appear, and it will really help you to see just why you need to eat or avoid certain foods.

Breaking the habit

In a nutshell, we eat what we eat out of habit. Old patterns of behaviour, usually rooted in childhood, are so ingrained and so familiar to us that they become totally automatic. So, if we are stressed we turn to cakes, biscuits or chocolate; when we wake up in the morning, we pour ourselves a bowl of cereal with milk; when we get to lunchtime, we have a cheese sandwich and a packet of crisps. Our present food choices are usually based on what we did in the past.

But what if what you eat (and what you fail to eat) is impacting negatively on your mood and health? What if your mood swings, depression, anxiety and poor concentration are directly linked to your diet? What if your diet is putting you at risk of disease?

Increasingly, research is confirming what nutritionists, dietitians and most ancient healing systems, such as Ayurveda and Traditional

Chinese Medicine (TCM), have known for a long time: that your thoughts, feelings and actions are intimately influenced by what you eat and drink. In fact, there is now good evidence to suggest that every aspect of you – body, health, libido, appearance, behaviour, sleep, motivation, vitality, ability to concentrate and even your IQ – is influenced, for better or for worse, by your diet. Getting your diet wrong, by eating the wrong ratios and amounts of macronutrients (carbohydrates, proteins and fats), foods to which you are allergic or intolerant or foods that are known to adversely affect mood – such as high-fructose corn syrup, sugar, trans-fatty acids, hydrogenated fats, additives, chemical contaminants – is increasingly being recognised as a major contributor to sub-optimal emotional, physical and mental health. Depression, anxiety, autism, mood swings, ADHD and Alzheimer's disease are just a handful of the diseases that are linked to poor nutrition.[21]

The healthy-eating challenge

The goal of my healthy-eating programme is to provide you with great-tasting food that contains the best forms of the macronutrients discussed above, sustains your energy and mood, meets the nutritional and energy requirements of your body, helps you to maintain your ideal weight, supports the process of healing and recovery from illness, reduces inflammation, prevents disease and optimises your physical, emotional and psychological potential. Or, put simply: to help you thrive and flourish.

However, a lot of what actually constitutes healthy eating depends on you. Your level of physical activity, rate of metabolism, lifestyle, life stage, nutrient and hormone levels and the presence of stress all influence what the optimum diet for you is. The food that's available, your preferences, your financial resources and the eating habits of your family are also relevant.

Create a personalised optimum nutrition plan

While I believe that most people would benefit from a diet that is tailored specially for them by a nutritional therapist or nutritionally trained health professional, they can, in my experience, create a pretty good nutrition programme by following the four steps that I recommend to my own patients and which I outline below.

- **Step 1** – Follow healthy-eating principles
- **Step 2** – Emphasise health-promoting foods
- **Step 3** – Avoid/limit health-depleting foods
- **Step 4** – Take supplements to support your health

Step 1: Follow healthy-eating principles

While health professionals, dietitians, doctors and nutritionists tend to differ in the finer details of what they think constitutes a healthy diet, there are some general healthy-eating principles that most agree upon on. The following was developed in conjunction with my nutritional therapist colleague Christine Bailey and provides the foundations upon which the remaining three steps are built.

Eat three meals and two snacks a day

One of the most important ways to be certain that your moods don't fluctuate is to ensure that your body and brain is provided with a stable supply of glucose (fuel) throughout the day. Eating three carbohydrate-containing meals and two snacks (one mid-morning and one mid-afternoon) a day, and eating protein with each of these, will help to prevent dips in the supply of blood sugar to the brain.

Avoid skipping meals

While skipping meals might seem tempting, especially if you are trying to lose weight, your brain will actually think that you are entering a period of starvation and it will automatically increase cravings for high-calorie foods. Missing meals places you at much greater risk of ultimately eating more calories and less healthy food at your next meal. It also increases the likelihood of blood-sugar dips and swings in your mood and energy.

Keep hydrated

Aim for between 2 and 3 litres of water a day. I've noticed that when I am dehydrated my clarity of thinking and mood decrease. I recommend either drinking filtered water or reverse-osmosis water (see Resources, page 281, for information).

Go organic

Because organic foods tend to contain fewer chemicals than non-organic, which may or may not contribute to health issues (the research is controversial), you might want to consider following the guidance provided by the Environmental Working Groups who suggest purchasing organic versions of those fruits and vegetables that are known to have, on average, the highest levels of pesticides.[22]

- Highest in pesticides: peaches, apples, peppers, celery, nectarines, strawberries, cherries, kale, lettuce, grapes (imported), carrots and pears

- Lowest in pesticides: onions, avocados, sweetcorn, pineapples, mangoes, asparagus, kiwi, cabbage, aubergines, watermelon, broccoli, tomatoes and sweet potatoes

Washing fruits and vegetables can also to help to reduce the pesticide load by a small amount. Wherever possible, choose locally sourced in-season produce.

When it comes to meat, my recommendation is to invest in quality, the gold standard being organic meat; this way, you avoid eating meat that may be laden with hormones, steroids and antibiotics. Another good alternative is grass-fed meat, which tends to be higher in healthy fats, such as omega-3s, conjugated linoleic acid and vitamins E and beta-carotene, and lower in total fat and calories.

Follow the 80/20 rule

Essentially, this rule says that if you make the majority (80 per cent) of what you eat health-promoting food, then, as long as you are essentially fit and well, you may eat what you like for the other 20 per cent (as long as you aren't intolerant to that food). The idea behind this is that it's important to be flexible when it comes to eating and that you don't enter a self-deprivation consciousness in which you get too uptight or restrictive about what you eat. And let's face it, there are some exquisite-tasting foods out there that are laden with sugar, but which should be enjoyed once in a while. It's a question of balance. That said, if you have a significant health issue, such as cancer, the split between healthy and unhealthy food needs to be nearer 90/10 or even 100 per cent healthy.

Eat until satisfied and then stop

Overeating can lead to and be a symptom of low self-esteem, stress and depression. Portion size and calorie intake therefore is an important part of healthy eating. Most women need about 2000 calories and men 2500 calories a day. Obviously men and women who are smaller and less physically active will need fewer, while larger and/or physically active people will need more. As a general rule of thumb, I encourage my patients to eat until they sense they are satisfied, to put their knife and fork down between mouthfuls, to eat off small plates, to eat soup (this keeps you feeling fuller for longer) and to choose smaller portion sizes, particularly when in a restaurant. Another good guide is to eat no more than would fit into your cupped hands.

Identify and address emotional eating

Emotional eating is a strategy that we use in order to change and improve the way we feel. You are probably an emotional eater if you regularly use food to manage stress, sadness, boredom, anger, fear, agitation, shame, guilt or frustration. You can have the best of intentions and all the knowledge you need about a healthy diet, but if you use food to manage your stress, it will almost certainly sabotage your healthy-eating programme. Following the advice in Pillars One and Two will help you to avoid this pitfall and to stay on track.

Step 2: Emphasise health-promoting foods

Now that you're familiar with the principles of healthy eating, here's a practical guide to the foods that you should emphasise in your diet.

Vegetables

Getting your recommended 'five a day' is an important part of ensuring good health (and preventing a wide variety of health problems, such as cancer and heart disease). A portion is about 80g of fruit or vegetables. This is roughly equal to: an apple, orange, banana or similarly sized fruit; two plums, nectarines or similarly sized fruit; a handful or grapes or berries; a slice of melon, pineapple or large fruit; one tablespoon of raisins or other dried fruit; two serving spoons of cooked vegetables; a dessert bowl of salad; two serving spoons of beans and pulses (this only counts for one portion a day); or a 150ml glass of fresh fruit juice or smoothie (only one portion a day). Wherever possible, eat a variety of in-season fruits and vegetables in order to benefit from their unique nutrient content. You should be aiming for a minimum of three portions of vegetables and two of fruit a day.

Carbohydrates

Carbohydrates provide the brain and body with glucose for fuel and energy. The key to good mental health is to eat low amounts of 'refined' carbohydrates (which tend to cause rapid swings in the blood-sugar level) and instead favour high-quality 'natural' carbohydrates. The latter, when broken down by the body, cause a more gentle, sustained release of glucose into the bloodstream, while also (unlike most refined carbohydrates) providing the brain and body with other valuable nutrients, such as fibre, minerals and vitamins. Eating natural carbohydrates helps to prevent the fluctuating supply of glucose that is associated with tiredness, mood swings, irritability, poor concentration and a reduction in mental performance.[23]

Here are some tips for eating the right carbohydrates:

- 'Natural' carbohydrates exist, as their name suggests, in their natural whole state. They include vegetables, oatmeal, wholegrain bread, beans, lentils, fruit, wholegrain pasta and wholegrain cereals. Wholegrains contain higher levels of fibre, protein and minerals such as potassium and selenium when compared with refined grains.

- The best wholegrains to eat are quinoa, cornmeal, oats, rye, barley, rice, millet, buckwheat, amaranth, kamut, spelt and wholewheat (as long as you are not intolerant to them). Aim for a minimum of three servings a day.

- Swap white for brown foods. For example, eat wholegrain breads, brown rice, basmati rice, wholewheat pasta and wholewheat noodles, rather than refined or processed starches (white bread, white rice and white pasta).

Protein/amino acids

Amino acids provide the building blocks for neuropeptides and neurotransmitter – the molecules of emotion that allow the cells and systems of your body and brain to communicate. I will be talking about neurotransmitters in some depth in Pillar Five (see page 126), but what you need to know here is that you must eat enough high-quality sources of protein (which is broken down by the process of digestion into amino acids) in order to ensure that the nerve cells in your brain and body are able to produce the relevant neurotransmitter type.

The best and healthiest sources of protein are organic or grass-fed lean meat, fish, seafood, eggs, beans, nuts, seeds, lentils, chickpeas, peas, hummus, tahini, nut butters (almond, hazelnut and sugar-free peanut butter), quinoa, cheese and yoghurt. Fermented soya products such as miso, tempeh and tamari are also good, but avoid processed forms of soya, such as TVP. Because red meat and dairy (two good sources of protein) can, when eaten in significant amounts, promote inflammation in the body, which is in itself associated with a variety of health problems, such as heart disease, Alzheimer's disease and cancer, red meat should be limited to twice a week and dairy either avoided or limited to one serving a day. If you choose dairy, my recommendation is to go for organic.

The amount of protein you need really does depend on you, as there are genetic, physical and metabolic factors to consider. As a general rule, however, most of us need to eat protein with each meal and snack, to help stabilise our blood sugar, as well as supply our body with amino acids, but the amount of protein needs to be worked out by you: if you have a strong appetite, would experience low energy levels after having just an orange or apple juice for breakfast and if you would find it hard to go without eating during the day, you probably need to have a quite high level of protein. Try experimenting with eating different levels of protein each day, varying between animal- and plant-based sources, and your body (through the way you feel and your energy levels) will tell you what's best.

Fats/Oils

While the word 'fat' gets a bad rap, because of the 'low-fat diet' movement, eating the right kinds of fat and avoiding the wrong kinds is essential to emotional health. The oils you use both on your food and in your cooking can, for example, have a significant impact on your health, mood and risk of developing disease later on in life. The best oil to use on your vegetables and salads is organic cold-pressed extra virgin oil.[24] It is rich in anti-inflammatory essential fatty acids and is regarded as being one of the main reasons why the Mediterranean diet has been shown to have so many positive benefits. Unrefined coconut oil is an excellent choice for cooking with, as it remains stable at higher temperatures, so when heated it doesn't create free radicals which damage our health, although olive oil is a good alternative. Low-salt butter tastes great on bread and on vegetables, but it is a saturated fat and should be eaten in moderation (as should other sources of saturated fats, as found in meat, dairy and eggs).[25]

Other healthy fats include monounsaturated fats, such as those found in olives and avocados, phospholipids and essential fatty acids (both of which are covered below).

Essential fatty acids (EFAs)

EFAs are fats that cannot be manufactured by the body, but are required to maintain optimum health. The two main types – omega-3 (alpha-linolenic) and omega-6 (linoleic) are required for almost every bodily function, including growth and repair, mood and memory, healthy cell membranes, immune function, hormonal balance, energy production, cardiovascular health and maintaining the health of skin, hair and nails, brain and nervous system.

Omega-3 and omega-6 work best together when taken in roughly equal amounts, however, for most people in the West the ratio tends to be closer to 1:6 and even 1:20 in some people. The excessive consumption of vegetable oils found in processed foods combined with a

34 per cent decline in vegetable consumption and a 59 per cent drop in fish intake in the last sixty years[26] (both good sources of omega-3) has led to this imbalance and this is thought to be a critical factor in a variety of diseases. One study, for example, compared 264 adults aged over sixty with depressive symptoms (including just over 100 with depressive disorders), with 461 randomly selected reference subjects. They used blood samples to measure concentrations of omega-3 and omega-6 fatty acids in the blood. Omega-3 fatty acids were significantly lower, and the ratio of omega-6 to omega-3 was higher in subjects with depressive disorders than in control subjects.[27] It is thought that low levels of dietary omega-3 are associated with low levels of the neuro-transmitter serotonin. A lack or imbalance of these EFAs has also been associated with schizophrenia, depression, attention deficit hyperactive disorder (ADHD), learning difficulties and behavioural problems.[28]

Good sources of omega-3 essential fatty acids include oily fish, such as wild Alaskan salmon, sardines, herring, kippers, anchovies, mackerel and trout (eat oily fish twice to three times a week); dark green leafy vegetables; flax seeds; and walnuts.

Good sources of omega-6 essential fatty acids include: sunflower, sesame, hemp and pumpkin seeds, evening primrose oil and borage oil.

Phospholipids

The phospholipids phosphatidyl choline, phosphatidyl serine and DMAE are a group of intelligent fats that play a very important role in memory, as well as mood, clear thinking and mental performance. In addition to forming the bulk of the myelin sheath which insulates the body's nerve cells (thus ensuring the smooth, quick flow of information around the brain and body), they allow the cells and systems of the body to communicate efficiently. Deficiencies are associated with poor memory, slow learning, difficulty concentrating, forgetfulness and declining memory.[29]

Good sources of phospholipids include eggs (organic, free-range), sardines and organ meats, such as liver and kidneys.

Step 3: Avoid/limit health-depleting foods

When it comes to emotional health and happiness, there are certain foods or ingredients within food that are known to have a negative impact on the way you feel, think and behave. In this step, I have listed those that you should consider reducing or preferably eliminating. For most of my patients with mood disorders, such as depression and anxiety, I recommend that they come off sugar, refined carbohydrates, caffeine and any foods to which they are intolerant for a two-week trial. The majority notice a positive shift in their well-being and mood, and some experience a complete transformation in the way they feel. Not everyone needs to do this, but some people do. To find out whether you are one of those people, I would highly recommend doing the two-week trial. If you crave sugar you might be sugar sensitive; if so, you can download an article from my website on the subject.

The following are the foods and drinks that I recommend you consider either limiting or eliminating in order to improve your emotional health:

Foods that you are intolerant or sensitive to

If you suffer from bloating, flatulence, constipation, diarrhoea, headaches, skin rashes, fatigue, cravings, fluid retention or facial puffiness, you should consider the possibility that you have a food intolerance or sensitivity.[30] The most common food intolerances are to cow's milk and cheese, wheat, gluten (found in wheat, rye, spelt, kamut, barley and oats – oats often contain gluten as a contaminant), corn, beef, yeast, eggs, garlic, peanuts, seeds, nightshade vegetables (tomatoes, potatoes, aubergines and peppers), kiwi and soya. If you have any of the symptoms above see the allergies/food intolerance section in Pillar Five for advice.

Refined carbohydrates

Refined carbohydrates are found in white bread, white pasta, rolls, pastry, cakes, biscuits, confectionery, carbonated drinks, fruit juice drinks and certain processed breakfast cereals. There is a lot of evidence linking the consumption of refined carbohydrates with obesity, heart disease, certain cancers, stroke, non-insulin dependent diabetes, atherosclerosis and a lower life expectancy.[31] The sugar lows they can create also adversely affect mood. Try to limit yourself to a maximum of three products per week.

Sugar

Apart from the various kinds of sugar we see on the supermarket shelves, sugar is an ingredient in a whole host of foods, including processed foods, soda, cereals, baked beans, sausages, beefburgers and even cheese. It also appears in the numerous guises, such as barley malt, brown rice syrup, corn syrup, date sugar, dextrin, dextrose, fructose, fruit juice concentrate, galactose, glucose, high-fructose corn syrup, lactose, maltodextrin, malted barley, maltose, mannitol, maple syrup, microcrystalline cellulose, molasses, polydextrose, sorbitol, sucrose – the list is endless! For most people, and in modest amounts, sugar doesn't pose a problem. However, excessive consumption of sugar is known to lead to symptoms such as irritability, mood swings, anxiety, aggressive behaviour, difficulty concentrating and depression.

In the long term, sugar and refined carbohydrates have been associated with a high level of inflammation of the body and brain, attention deficit hyperactive disorder (ADHD), suppression of the immune system, lower IQ, premenstrual syndrome, obesity, tooth decay, osteoporosis, heart disease, metabolic syndrome, Alzheimer's disease, diabetes, cancer and age-related macular degeneration.[32] I encourage the majority of my patients to significantly reduce the amount of sugar they consume.

Trans-fatty acids

These are found in crisps, biscuits, crackers, doughnuts, margarines, vegetable shortening, baked goods, French fries, fried foods, snack foods and most processed foods. Trans-fats are created by the hydrogenation of vegetable oil – a process that gives the oil a longer shelf life and makes it more solid at room temperature. These damaged fats are also linked to heart disease, insulin resistance and Alzheimer's disease.[33] Trans-fatty acids should be avoided altogether.

Sweeteners

These are found in Nutrasweet, Equal and Spoonful, among others and should be avoided altogether. There is an increasing body of evidence linking the regular consumption of sweeteners to mental agitation, headaches, depression, lowered seizure threshold and even cancer.[34] I'd recommend you consider using the sugar substitute xylitol, which is a natural sweetener that not only has a minimal negative impact on blood-sugar levels but has also been found to reduce tooth decay and the risk of middle-ear infections.

Caffeine

Caffeine is one of the world's most popular stimulants. It is found in over sixty different species of plants and is most commonly ingested in coffee, tea, cola, soft drinks, chocolate and pick-me-up tablets. While for many people a couple of cups of tea or coffee has no negative impact on mood or health, for others it very much does.

One way to find out how caffeine is affecting you is to come off it and see if you have any withdrawal symptoms. I recommend doing this if you drink more than one cup of coffee, two cups of tea, two cans of caffeinated drink (Pepsi, Coke, Diet Coke or Red Bull, for example) or three cups of green tea or Earl Grey tea a day. Excess consumption of caffeine has been associated with caffeine dependency, mood swings, blood-sugar instability, anxiety, depression, irritability, tiredness, headaches, adrenal fatigue, endometriosis, mineral deficiencies and fibroids.[35]

When coming off caffeine, and especially if you are consuming more than 300mg a day (equivalent to three cups of instant coffee), you might want to consider reducing your caffeine consumption by half each day until you reach zero. If you get any withdrawal symptoms (tiredness, headaches, irritability and mood fluctuations), keep yourself hydrated with water and consider taking the amino acid l-tyrosine (1000mg twice a day) – this will help to reduce the symptoms. They should disappear naturally within two to nine days of stopping caffeine.

I'd recommend you avoid caffeine altogether or limit consumption to less than 300mg a day.

Alcohol

Most people can drink moderate amounts of alcohol without it being detrimental to their health. Indeed, there might even be an overall benefit to the heart, but this needs to be balanced with an increased risk of developing cancer. Also, the evidence is pretty strong now that if you are attempting to have a baby, you should stop all alcohol and remain alcohol-free throughout the pregnancy and breastfeeding period.

In my experience of patients who have an unhealthy relationship with alcohol, most of those who habitually use it in the evening are simply using it to medicate feelings of stress and tension, while others have a dependence on it. This really needs to be diagnosed by a professional trained in the assessment and treatment of addictions, but broadly speaking, if you answer 'Yes' to one of the following, it is an indication that you should seek advice:

- Have you ever felt you should cut down on your drinking?

- Have people ever annoyed you by criticising your drinking?

- Have you ever felt bad or guilty about your drinking?

- Have you ever had a drink first thing in the morning (an 'eye-opener') to steady your nerves or get rid of a hangover?

If you have insomnia, candida, cancer, an immune or autoimmune system problem, or are simply dedicated to experiencing your full health and well-being potential you should consider reducing your intake or coming off alcohol completely. The latter is preferable, not just because of the physical benefits, but also because of the emotional ones. Couples, for example, are much more likely to interact meaningfully when they are not drinking alcohol. Plus, alcohol-free evenings provide the time and space to do what you really enjoy. With a couple of exceptions, the people and patients who I consider to be enjoying the highest levels of health and fulfilment are those who don't drink alcohol.

I'd recommend that you avoid alcohol or limit your consumption to two units (for women) or three (for men) a day.

Step 4: Take supplements to support your health

It would be nice to think that we could get all the vitamins, minerals, antioxidants and healthy fats we need from our diet, but in reality we can't and don't.

In the UK, the Food Standards Agency survey tells us the average adult male is consuming just 2.7 portions of fruit and vegetables on average, while the average adult female consumes 2.9.[36] What's more, the fruit and vegetables that we do eat vary enormously in their nutrient content, depending on where they were grown; overall, when compared with their equivalents fifty years ago, they contain between 10 and 70 per cent fewer essential minerals.[37] Another study found that women are particularly lacking in essential minerals, with more than 91 per cent not getting their reference nutrient intake (RNI) of iron (14.8mg), more than 74 per cent not getting their RNI of magnesium (270mg) and almost 50 per cent not getting their RNI of calcium (700mg). In addition, nearly half of men are not getting their RNI of magnesium and one in three men is not getting his RNI of zinc, which is considered to play an important role in mental health and motivation.[38]

Put simply, to help us reach our emotional health potential, we all need to supplement our diets.

Which supplements should you take?

Supplements are a very personal thing, and it really does depend on you, your health and budget as to which supplements you choose. In an ideal world you'd get a nutritionist or integrative medical doctor to run tests to identify which nutrients you are deficient in and then have a programme developed around that. But that costs money, and the accuracy of some tests is unknown. Therefore, as a general rule, I recommend:

- A multivitamin–mineral supplement
- Vitamin C with bioflavonoids
- Essential fatty acids
- Probiotics
- Additional minerals (according to need)

This might sound like a lot of supplements and understandably you might be concerned about the cost. My take on supplements is that they are an investment in your health and that the pound or so a day (which is what these will cost in total) is worth it. If your budget is very tight I recommend prioritising the multivitamin–mineral and essential fatty acid supplements.

THE IMPORTANCE OF VITAMINS AND MINERALS

Most of us know that we need vitamins and minerals for good health and well-being. But not everyone knows why. Here are just a few facts and figures to illustrate the importance of getting your vitamin and mineral balance right:

- Deficiencies of vitamin C, various B vitamins, folic acid, magnesium and zinc are associated with an increased incidence and severity of depression.[39]

- Magnesium is required for over 300 different enzyme reactions in your body and is essential for energy production and strengthening your bones and teeth. Magnesium deficiency is associated with depression, anxiety, tension, insomnia, ADHD, irritability, muscle cramps, premenstrual syndrome (PMS) mood changes, noise sensitivity and autism.[40]

- Zinc deficiency is associated with eating disorders, lack of motivation, depression and loss of appetite. [41]

- One study found that between 15 and 38 per cent of people with depression have low folic acid levels in their bodies and those with very low levels tend to be the most depressed.[42]

- B vitamins, especially B_6, B_{12} and folic acid are essential for a process called methylation, which is needed to keep your hormones and neurotransmitters in balance. Adequate levels of the B vitamins are also critical for optimum energy levels, mental performance and memory. [43]

Multivitamin–mineral supplements

Getting the right amounts and ratios of vitamins and minerals is an essential component of and contributor to your emotional health and happiness. The dosages below are intended only as a guide to the levels of nutrients that you should look for in a multivitamin–mineral–antioxidant supplement. The exact amount, however, depends on your sex, age, level of activity, health and your health and well-being goals.

For emotional health most people will need to take supplements that provide a daily total dose in the region of:

- Vitamin A: 5000–10,000IU (avoid if pregnant)

- Mixed carotenoids: 2500–25,000IU

- Vitamin D$_3$: 400–1000IU

- Vitamin C: 200–1000mg

- Mixed tocopherols: 400IU or vitamin E – 100–400IU

- Vitamin B: B$_1$ – 25–100mg; B$_2$ – 25–100mg; B$_3$ – 50–100mg; B$_5$ – 25–100mg; B$_6$ – 25–100mg; B$_{12}$ – 10–1000mcg

- Biotin: 50–300mcg

- Choline: 20–100mg

- Folic acid: 400–1000mcg

- Inositol: 20–300 mg

- Calcium: 600–800mg

- Magnesium: 400–600mg

- Chromium: 100–400 mcg

- Iodine: 25–75mcg

- Boron: 0.5–5mg

- Copper: 1mg

- Manganese: 1–10mg

- Selenium: 25–100mcg

- Zinc: 10–30mg

- and possibly others, such molybdenum, potassium, and vitamin K

Note: iron (5 to 15mg) should, as a general rule, only be taken if you are known to be deficient in it or at risk of deficiency. Most menstruating women will need it.

Quite a few of the vitamins and minerals listed above, such as vitamins D and C, calcium and magnesium, will need to be taken as a separate supplement in order to achieve the optimal dosage. In practice this means you will probably need to take about six tablets/capsules a day, in addition to your essential fatty acids and probiotic supplements.

Vitamin C 1000mg with bioflavonoids

Because vitamin C is quite bulky, most multivitamins won't supply the preferred amount. You should therefore consider taking a vitamin C supplement. Both vitamin C and bioflavonoids are potent antioxidants and anti-inflammatory supplements and are required to ensure optimum levels of the brain's neurotransmitters.

Essential fatty acids

We have already seen how important omega-3 and omega-6 essential fatty acids are for your emotional health. Most people will benefit from taking 1000mg to 2000mg of fish oil initially (or flaxseed oil for vegetarians), for a couple of months, in order to restore a healthy ratio and balance between the two essential fatty acids. Make sure you choose a fish oil product that is guaranteed to be free of mercury, PCBs (polychlorinated biphenyls) and other pollutants. After this, you should consider switching to either a formula that provides EPA and DHA (all of these are omega-3 EFAs) and GLA (the omega-6 essential fatty acid) or continue with your fish oil or flaxseed oil and supplement with 1000mg to 4000mg of GLA-rich oils, such as borage oil (contains 24 per cent GLA), evening primrose oil (8 per cent) or blackcurrant oil (15 per cent); follow the manufacturers' recommendations for dosage.

If you have a mental-health problem or any of the classic symptoms of omega-3 deficiency (fatigue, dry and/or itchy skin – including goose-bump rash on the upper arms and/or upper thighs – excessive thirst, sweating or urination), brittle hair and nails, constipation, frequent infections, PMS, depression, poor concentration or memory, lack of physical endurance, and/or joint pain, you should consider upping your dose of fish oil to between 3000mg and 10,000mg a day.

Probiotics

Probiotics, from the Greek, 'for life', refers to over 400 strains of bacteria that naturally reside within our intestines. Because of poor diet, stress, alcohol and the overuse of certain medications, most people have a degree of digestive imbalance and will benefit from taking a high-quality probiotic supplement. (See Dysbiosis in Pillar Five, page 168, for more information.)

While there are many different types of probiotic, you should look for one that contains a variety of synergistic probiotic strains including lactobacilli and bifidobacteria. The total daily dose should be in the region of 10 billion viable organisms. You might need more if you have a specific gut problem.

Minerals

A healthy diet and a multivitamin–mineral supplement will ensure that you receive most of the vitamins and minerals that you need. However, I tend to find that a number of my patients, especially those with a chronic health challenge need additional minerals as well. Deficiencies of many of the essential minerals, including zinc, magnesium and calcium are more common than deficiencies of vitamins, because the body doesn't manufacture minerals. Many of the soils within which our fruits and vegetables grow are depleted in minerals, and this, in turn, makes for mineral-depleted produce. And while organic produce does tend to have higher levels, these are fairly modest increases in the range of 5 to 15 per cent.

To work out which minerals you need to take, you can either have a blood test (which can be expensive and obviously invasive) or you can use a mineral test kit (see Resources, page 282). Although research relating to the use of these kits is limited (the exception being the zinc taste test[44]), my patients have found them to be a very useful way of helping them to adjust the types and levels of minerals that they take.

Get active

Daily physical activity is essential for the health of your mind, the quality of your mood and the prevention of future health-related problems. What's more, regular physical activity can help to release stored psychological and emotional tension, increase stress resilience, stimulate the production of new brain cells and inter-brain cell connections, increase feelings of self-worth and self-confidence, balance hormones, prevent and stabilise insulin resistance, reduce body fat, increase bone mass and reduce the risk of heart disease, stroke, hip fractures and breast cancer.[45]

As you can see, exercise is a very good thing! One study compared the effectiveness of exercise alone, versus medication alone and versus medication plus exercise in relieving the symptoms of people with major depressive disorders. After four and a half months of treatment, patients receiving all three of these treatments were significantly less depressed, while about two-thirds were no longer depressed. Six months after the study concluded, the patients were followed up. Researchers found that patients who had been in the exercise group were more likely to be partially or fully recovered than those who were in the medication or medication plus exercise group.[46]

While most of us know that we would benefit from more physical activity, in reality we struggle to get enough of it. But the good news is that with a bit of motivation, a little knowledge and some forward planning that can all change.

What counts as physical activity?

Physical activity includes, among other things, jogging, swimming, brisk walking, rebounding (using a mini-trampoline), climbing stairs, yoga, Pilates, cycling, gardening (weeding, mowing, raking), vacuuming, sweeping, dancing, playing golf, painting, decorating and, of course, sex.

The key, as far as emotional health and happiness is concerned, is to include a variety that covers the three main types of exercise:

1. **Aerobic training** This helps to improve the health of the heart and circulation system and to maintain optimum weight. Examples include jogging, brisk walking, cycling, swimming or rebounding.

2. **Strength-training** This increases your metabolic rate (and, therefore, helps with weight loss), improves muscle strength and co-ordination and prevents osteoporosis. Examples include weight-training, climbing stairs, push-ups, sit-ups, using resistance bands and cycling.

3. **Flexibility or stretching exercises** These improve overall range of movement, mobility and co-ordination. These exercises can also help to release muscular and emotional tension. Examples include yoga, t'ai chi and Pilates.

Tips for improving your physical activity level and fitness

Note: as a general rule, if you are over the age of fifty, haven't exercised before or have a serious or debilitating medical condition you must always get the green light to go ahead from your GP before exercising, and have an exercise programme prescribed for you by someone who is trained to provide one.

Get motivated

Most people don't exercise regularly because they haven't made it a priority in their lives and because they haven't yet established exercise as a habit. Here are some suggestions to get you motivated:

- Partner up with a motivated friend.

- Write down a list of the potential benefits to you of exercising.

- Join *and* attend (this is the most important bit!) a running, cycling, swimming or similar activity-based club.

- Employ a personal trainer.

- Commit to walking/running on behalf of a charity.

Choose your physical activities

Make a list of all of the physical activities that you could realistically do. Include a mix of the three types of exercise outlined above.

Honour your body and fitness level

If you haven't exercised for a while, start gradually with walking, increasing to brisk walking, then jogging and, if you are fit enough, running. Most gyms have personal trainers who will create a tailored programme for you. Consider this as an option, particularly if lack of motivation or inexperience are factors for you.

Aim for between thirty and forty-five minutes of physical activity daily

If you can't manage this daily, start with three times a week and take it from there. It's important to set yourself a realistic target. The UK government recommends a minimum of thirty minutes for adults and sixty minutes for children of moderate-intensity physical activity on at least five days of the week. You can also work exercise into your daily routine by parking further away from the office and walking to work, for example, or taking the stairs instead of a lift or escalator. A useful way to monitor this is to use a pedometer – the target for most people is 10,000 steps a day.

Plan the week ahead in a diary

Write down the activities you are going to do and on which days. For example: Monday – brisk walk to and from work; Tuesday – swim after work; Wednesday – yoga after work; Thursday – brisk walk to and from work; Friday – weight-training and push-ups before work; Saturday – gardening; Sunday – walk in the countryside with family.

Try the talk test

When doing aerobic exercise you should aim for moderate intensity. One way to gauge this is with the 'talk test': exercise hard enough to break into a sweat, but not so hard that you can't carry on a conversation.

Exercise mindfully

When you do any physical activity, try keeping your full attention within your body, focus on your breathing and relax into the movements of your body. This will help you to enjoy it more and it will improve your performance.

Sleep soundly

Think back to a time recently when you didn't have a good night's sleep. How did it impact on the following day? Did it affect your mood or decision-making ability? How did it impact on your choice of food and drink? Were you more or less likely to exercise or eat sugary snacks?

For most people, having one or more disturbed night's sleep will have an obvious negative impact on their mood and decisions. But what if sleep deprivation was an ongoing problem – what impact would this have?

A survey carried out by the National Sleep Foundation in 2005 revealed how serious and widespread a problem sleep deprivation is. About 40 per cent of people get fewer than seven hours sleep on weekdays, while 70 per cent get fewer than eight.[47] Sleep deprivation is a way of life for most people. Those most likely to be at risk include commuters, people under stress or suffering anxiety, those who work long hours and/or spend a long time in their car, parents with small children and, of course, insomniacs.

Sleep and your health

Sleep deprivation, which is an acute or chronic lack of sufficient restorative sleep, puts you at a higher risk of developing heart disease and cancer, but has also been shown to promote weight gain, exacerbate and trigger depression and anxiety, reduce immune function and increase the likelihood of accidents.[48] Sleep deprivation also puts you at much higher risk of making poor health choices and life decisions. For example, a poll organised by the National Sleep Foundation in America found that 80 per cent of women managed to fight through the daytime tiredness associated with sleep deprivation by drinking caffeine-rich drinks, with one third admitting they consumed three or more such drinks every day in an attempt to escape their exhaustion. Half the women confessed that they sacrifice exercise and, in addition, more than a third said they also reduce the amount of time spent with friends and family, stop eating healthily and don't participate in sexual activity when feeling tired.[49] Sleep deprivation affects every level and aspect of your life.

Tips for improving your sleep

Here are some practical ideas to help you get more – and better quality – sleep.

Identify and address the cause of your sleep problem

Perhaps you are having difficulty sleeping because of stress, for example, or your hormones, your inability to fully relax before bed or your physical environment? Wherever possible, take action to address those causes. You might want to use blackout blinds in your room to keep it dark or try a stress-reduction approach prior to bed.

Also, watch the temperature of your room. Try to keep it at a slightly cool setting, as this will help you get to sleep and to achieve a deeper level of sleep – 18–21°C (65–70°F) is the ideal temperature.

Avoid stimulants and stimulating experiences

If you have problems sleeping, you might want try cutting out all caffeine during the day (or at least not having any after 4 p.m.) and reducing your intake of sugar, especially in the hours leading up to bedtime. Nicotine is also stimulating – if you are a smoker, try to avoid smoking prior to bedtime. Potentially stimulating experiences, such as TV, work, checking e-mails and being on the Internet should also be avoided for at least three hours prior to bedtime. If you have a TV in your room I highly recommend you take it out; keep your room for sleep and sexual intimacy.

Avoid medications that interfere with sleep

The main ones are cough and cold remedies that contain phenylephrine and pseudoephedrine, painkillers and tablets containing caffeine, steroids and stimulants, such as Ritalin and antihistamines. I would also really encourage you to steer clear of benzodiazepines (sleeping tablets). While they do help the short term, they can lead to dependency in the longer term. My advice would be to use these only as a last resort, after trying the rest of my recommendations.

If you need something to help you sleep, try natural sleep remedies; the ones I use most often with my patients are valerian (follow manufacturer's instructions), magnesium (400–500mg) or the nutrient 5-HTP (100–200mg) at bedtime.

Also, if you regularly have trouble sleeping just prior to your period, try taking vitamin B_6 (100mg at bedtime). This helps to make the calming brain chemical serotonin. Take this with an additional vitamin B complex.

Get physical

You should be aiming for about thirty minutes of physical activity on most days (see page 113); this helps to discharge stress and tension. Avoid exercising in the evening though as it can be too stimulating.

Avoid eating heavy meals and avoid or limit alcohol

If you eat just before you go to bed, your body will be busy digesting and won't want to go to sleep, so leave a gap of at least two hours between a meal and bed.

While many insomniacs use alcohol to help them sleep, research shows that alcohol consumption prior to bed results in multiple awakenings, shallow sleep, a reduction in sleep time and overall quality. My advice is to steer clear of it.

Try guided imagery

Many of my patients with insomnia find that listening to a guided imagery insomnia CD prior to going to sleep is very helpful. (See Resources, page 281, for details.)

Relax your body and establish a good sleep routine

Remember your mind and body are intimately connected, so relaxing your body can really help to calm your mind prior to bedtime. Try having a hot, relaxing bath (with aromatherapy or alkaline mineral salts) and/or going to bed with a hot-water bottle.

Use everything you have learnt so far to establish a good sleeping pattern. Try to get to sleep by 10–10.30 p.m. and aim for about eight hours of sleep on most nights – this is enough for most people.

Create a negative association with waking up

If you are still awake after twenty minutes of attempting to sleep, get up and do something that you really don't enjoy doing, such as cleaning. This sets up a negative conditioning pattern that associates not sleeping with discomfort. By doing this, you are training your brain to help you get to sleep. One caveat: make sure you keep the lighting dim, as turning on the light tells your brain that it's time to wake up.

Use your tools

The two tools I find most helpful for insomnia are the emotional-processing tools, EmoTrance (page 53) and Cradling (page 55).

Seeking professional help

If you have insomnia that doesn't respond to any of the above measures or you experience excessive daytime sleepiness, abrupt awakening during the night, accompanied by shortness of breath, a morning headache, or you wake up with a dry mouth or sore throat, I'd encourage you to seek the help of a sleep specialist. These symptoms might indicate the presence of a serious sleep disorder called sleep apnoea.

Rest and relax

While most of us tend to be pretty good at keeping busy and mentally active, balancing this with rest and relaxation can be a real challenge.

Rest

Rest means not doing. It's about having unstructured 'empty' periods in your life, ideally on a daily basis. This is, of course, an unfamiliar experience for most of us, since we tend to rush from one thing to another, constantly filling our time with 'stuff'. But rest is designed to keep a check on that, to prevent us from getting too absorbed in doing and to help us cross over from 'doing' to 'being'.

During rest or empty time, you have no intentions, expectations or plans whatsoever – this is the key. You essentially trust and stay with the present moment and allow yourself to be guided by the creative impulse of the moment.

One thing to be aware of is that often the 'doing' mind will attempt to regain control and make suggestions for you. For example, you might have a thought to watch TV or call a friend. As a general rule, if an activity stimulates you, emotionally arouses you, increases tension or reduces your inner sense of calm then that is not rest. What actually happens during this empty time will really depend on you; what nourishes you might be very different for another person. Rest for me can sometimes be simply going for a walk, daydreaming, watching, lying on the grass, writing something or just simply sitting. I go with the moment and allow it to take me. If I get a thought, which I often do, of cutting short my rest period, I just notice it, let go of it and return my attention to the moment. In my experience, introducing regular periods of rest can help not only to rejuvenate the body and mind, but, as importantly, to open up channels of creativity and insight.

Tips for rest

- Try a seven-day experiment in which you commit to giving yourself some empty time each day. The exact length will depend on what works for you, but you should aim for ten minutes plus. Write these times into your diary and remember not to fill them with anything! I have found that this seven-day approach works well for my patients in terms of motivating them to try it, but if seven days sounds too much, go for three.

- Find a label for your rest period that gives it personal significance and meaning. Call it, for example, 'me time', 'quiet time' or 'prayer time'.

- Make sure you won't be disturbed during your rest time. Of course this is not easy if you have children.

- An attitude of playfulness, openness and curiosity can help the 'rest' process.

- Start your rest time by sitting still and focusing on your breath. When you get a thought to do something, ask yourself, 'Will this increase my sense of calm and nurture me from within?' If the answer is 'Yes', allow yourself to do it. If not, just wait patiently and something will come. If your 'doing' mind kicks in, or if you start judging yourself or your experience, just gently turn your attention back to the present moment.

- Whatever happens, allow yourself to enjoy the experience.

- Once your rest period is finished, reflect on your experience and how you are feeling. What did you learn about yourself? What insights did you get? How enjoyable was it? How motivated are you to give yourself another rest period?

Relaxation

Unlike rest, in which you allow the moment to direct your activities, relaxation is an active process designed to trigger a specific physiological response called the relaxation response (see below). Learning how to relax deeply and allow accumulated stress and tension to dissolve not only feels great, but is also an essential part of keeping healthy. Regular relaxation can help you manage stress, reduce levels of pain and discomfort, increase wound healing and even help you to access greater creativity.[50]

What is relaxation?

When I talk to my patients about relaxation, there appears to be quite a lot of confusion surrounding what counts as relaxation and what doesn't. So here are some guidelines to help you out; in order for something to qualify as relaxation the following four criteria need to be fulfilled:

1. It should have no adverse effects on your health, so smoking, drugs and alcohol do not count.

2. It should trigger your body's in-built physiological mechanism called the relaxation response. Essentially, this is designed to return the body to a place of balance. Signs that indicate it has been triggered include: feeling calm, relaxed and more connected to your surroundings; a decrease in your heart rate; relaxation of your muscles; and a deepening and slowing of your breathing.

3. You need to allow yourself to be present to whatever your relaxation activity is. For example, if your mind is distracted or you are not able to enjoy the experience, it doesn't count as relaxation. So a massage is relaxing only if you allow yourself to relax and enjoy it.

4. It should be something that fits in with you; everyone has different tastes and preferences. Going for a walk in the countryside could be deeply relaxing for one person, but boring or unpleasant for another.

Tips for relaxation

- As for rest, see if you can build a relaxation period into your daily routine. I recommend between fifteen and thirty minutes each day.

- Choose a couple of relaxation practices and try them out to discover which works for you. They include, among others, meditation, yoga, qigong, walking in nature, massage, taking a hot bath, listening to music, progressive muscle relaxation, prayer, mantras, hypnotherapy, conscious breathing, biofeedback and visualisation.

- Learn about stress management (see Pillar Six).

- Use guided imagery (see the exercise below).

EXERCISE: Body–mind relaxation

Try the following deep relaxation exercise:

- Find a quiet warm place where you will be undisturbed. Put on some relaxation music if you feel that might help you.

- Choose a word or phrase that you associate with relaxation. The key is that it should be meaningful to you and evoke feelings of calm and relaxation. For example, 'peace' or 'love'.

- Sit relaxed, close your eyes lightly and, keeping your eyes closed, 'look out' between your eyebrows. Breathe in and out through your nose.

- Imagine yourself in a place that you associate with being deeply relaxed. It could be somewhere you've been before or you can make up a place. Take a couple of deep breaths and allow yourself to feel at peace in this place.

- Now mentally scan your body for tension. Start at the top of the head and work your way down to your feet. If you locate any tension, deliberately increase that tension by contracting and tensing the relevant muscles. Bring it to its maximum intensity, then let it go suddenly and completely. Repeat this, paying particular attention to areas of the face and shoulders, which carry most of the body's tension. Take as long as you need to do this.

- Now say your key word on the out-breath and gently repeat it on each subsequent out-breath. If your mind strays or if you start judging yourself or your experience, just notice what has happened and gently return your attention back to the word and the breath. Continue with this for five to twenty minutes.

- Now – and this is optional – turn your attention to your feet. Imagine and feel your feet filling up with a white, rejuvenating energy. Feel and/or see its warmth as it circulates around your feet, dissolving as it does so, all stress, all tension and all discomfort.

- See and feel that bright white energy slowly rise in a spiralling fashion up into both ankles. As you breathe in, allow it to rise up higher into your calves, your knees and on up into the thighs. When it reaches the base of your spine, also feel and see it at your fingertips, ascending slowly into the fingers, the wrists, the fore-arms, the elbows, the upper arms and finally into the shoulders themselves. All the while, the warm energy continues rising up the spine, abdomen and chest until it meets the energy from your shoulders at your neck. Allow it to continue up the front, back and side of the head and all the way to the top. Wait a moment, return your attention to your breathing and enjoy the peace that follows.

- Once all tension has been dissolved, imagine a shower of bright white energy pouring down from the top of your head, descending to the neck, the shoulders and to the area of your heart, and from there spilling out into and around the body. Picture yourself within a sea of bright white light. Allow yourself as much time as you wish to enjoy this relaxed state.

Live and work in a healthy environment

Your environment has a major impact on your mood, emotional health and happiness. That might not come as a surprise; we all know how uplifting it can be when we go on holiday or for a walk in the country. Spending ten to fifteen minutes in natural sunlight a day has been shown to have numerous health benefits, not least that it triggers the creation of vitamin D within our bodies (indeed for many people it's their main source). Vitamin D deficiency is associated not only with depression,[51] but also with irritability, hyperactivity, apathy, seasonal affective disorder (SAD) and the presence of severe depressive symptoms (i.e. if you have depression and have vitamin D – sunlight – deficiency, the chances are that your symptoms will be worse when compared to someone who is not deficient). A study published in 2009 examined people aged sixty-five and over and found that those with the lowest levels of vitamin D were more than twice as likely as those with the highest levels of vitamin D to have problems with memory, attention, reasoning and judgement.[52]

Why is our environment so important?

For the last forty years, evidence has increasingly been emerging to confirm that our environment is saturated with toxins and chemicals from personal-care products, household products and building materials which, as well as air, food and water, have the potential to impact negatively on our heath and mood.

While many manufacturers claim that the chemicals within their products are not present in sufficient levels to cause harm (which is probably true in most cases), the concern relates both to their cumulative effects and to the potentially hazardous interactions between the various chemicals that we take into our bodies. And there is good cause for concern, since the presence of chemical toxins in the body is linked to a wide range of conditions, including autism, attention deficit hyperactive disorder (ADHD), chronic fatigue syndrome (CFS), multiple chemical sensitivities, multiple sclerosis, memory loss, childhood cancers, premature puberty, low sperm counts, testicular cancer, breast cancer, undescended testicles, multiple myeloma, non-Hodgkin's lymphoma, infertility, birth defects, asthma and learning disabilities.[53]

My own perspective on the issue of toxins and the environment is that until conclusive evidence is available, I recommend a precautionary approach which limits exposure to sources of harmful toxins, while doing everything possible to support the detoxification mechanisms of the body and liver through healthy eating and lifestyle changes.

Tips for a healthy environment

The following are some suggestions to help you limit your exposure to toxic influences and to enhance your environment, so that it supports and lifts your emotional health.

Surround yourself with beauty

Consider placing one or more objects or items of beauty in each room of your home – something that captures your eye and lifts your spirits every time you see it. This could be anything from plants and flowers to pictures, ornaments and sculptures. However, avoid having a cluttered home, as this will drain your energy.

Get outside

Most of us living in the UK are sun-starved, despite the fact that sunlight is an essential nutrient. Make sure you get at least ten to fifteen minutes in natural sunlight a day without sunscreen or sunglasses. You might also want to consider replacing some of your light bulbs with full-spectrum lighting (see Resources, page 281).

Avoid toxic personal-care and cleaning products

Try to use non-toxic personal-care and cleaning products. Deodorants, tampons, moisturisers, lipstick, hair dye, nail polish, perfumes and shower gels are made from chemicals, many of which are known carcinogens, allergens and hormone disruptors. Fortunately, there is now an increasing number of companies specialising in non-toxic personal-care products (see Resources, page 281).

Reduce your exposure to electromagnetic pollution

One of the unseen threats to our health is that posed by electromagnetic pollution. Our bodies are being bombarded with EMFs (electromagnetic frequencies) and ELFs (extremely low frequencies) from numerous different sources, such as computers, Wi-Fi, telephones, mobile phones, power lines, cell-phone relays, transformers, radios, radio transmitters, televisions and microwave ovens. While there is, to my knowledge, no absolute proof that these cause specific diseases, there is emerging evidence that they are a source of strain on the body. Mobile phones, for example, when used frequently and for long periods of time, can modify and damage certain structures in the brain.[54] There is, at present, very little evidence available to guide us on what constitutes a safe level of exposure and even less evidence on the long-term effects of electromagnetic pollution. So, until we know more, the advice I give to my patients is to play safe by making some simple adjustments:

- Limit the use of your mobile phone; use a land line whenever possible. Avoid placing your phone on your belt or in your top pocket, turn it off when not required and keep it away from the side of your bed when you are sleeping.

- Stay a minimum of 45 cm away from television and computer screens. Turn them off when not in use.

- Buy a cactus plant – *Cereus peruvianus* naturally restores an electromagnetically disturbed environment back to near normality.

- Move all electric clocks, clock radios and telephone answering machines at least 120 cm away from the head of the bed.

- Avoid using electric blankets, microwaves and hairdryers.

- Don't let your children play near power lines, transformers, radar domes and microwave towers.

PILLAR FOUR: Summary

- Meeting the physical needs of healthy diet, physical activity, sleep, rest, relaxation, sunlight and a healthy environment is an essential part of creating emotional health and happiness.

- The way you think and feel is intimately linked to the food you do and don't eat.

- Eating a healthy diet, rich in nutrient-dense whole foods and low in sugar, caffeine, processed foods and foods to which you are intolerant can lift your mood and help to transform your health.

Pillar Five: Identify and address physical imbalances

A significant proportion of my patients (about 80 per cent) have one or more physical imbalances that contribute to mood disturbances, preventing them from experiencing their full potential for emotional health and true happiness. What's more, evidence now points increasingly to the fact that for some people, their depression, irritability, anxiety, poor concentration, anger problems or ADHD are primarily related to imbalances affecting their physical body and brain.

In this pillar we are going to focus on five physical imbalances – the ones that I most commonly come across with my own patients:

- Neurotransmitter imbalances

- Nutritional imbalances

- Allergies and intolerances

- Hormone imbalances

- Dysbiosis

In the next few pages, you'll find the same physical-imbalance questionnaires that I use with my patients. They aren't diagnostic as such, but a score of 12 or more on any of them is a strong indication that there might be an issue that is preventing you from experiencing your full potential for true happiness and contributing to any signs and symptoms of mental distress that you have. Each question refers to the period of the last month. So, for the question 'Do you suffer from interrupted sleep or insomnia?', for example, you would answer 'Yes' if you had a problem three weeks ago, but not now.

Physical imbalance questionnaires

Neurotransmitter imbalances

Neurotransmitters are the chemical messengers of the nervous system. They relay information around and between the brain and the body. Although there are many different types of neurotransmitter that can affect your mood, I screen my patients for four of the most common ones: serotonin, GABA, acetylcholine and dopamine.

Take your time reading through the questionnaires. Read each question in turn, then score it as follows:

No = 0, Occasionally = 1, Yes = 2

If you answer 'Yes' to a question where you see an instruction in brackets, follow those instructions. Once you have added up your scores for each questionnaire, insert your totals in the score chart on page 137 or in your notebook or journal.

NEUROTRANSMITTER IMBALANCE QUESTIONNAIRES

Low serotonin levels

Do you:

- Experience obsessive behaviour or have difficulty in being flexible? (multiply your score by 2) ☐

- Experience irritability, restlessness, impatience, edginess or PMS? (multiply your score by 2) ☐

- Have a tendency to be negative, pessimistic and/or experience depression? ☐

- Have aggressive or suicidal thoughts? ☐

- Have repetitive, angry, guilty or self-critical thoughts? ☐

- Have feelings of low self-esteem and confidence? ☐

- Find it difficult to get to sleep or stay asleep? ☐

- Have a tendency to be fearful or shy? ☐

- Crave sugar, carbohydrates, salt and/or alcohol? ☐
- Feel worse in and dislike dark or hot weather? ☐

Total score ☐

Low GABA Levels

Do you:

- Experience anxiety or nervousness?
  (multiply your score by 2) ☐
- Feel unable to relax? (multiply your score by 2) ☐
- Get easily overwhelmed? (multiply your score by 2) ☐
- Have stiff and tense muscles? ☐
- Have a tendency to get paranoid or panicked? ☐
- Use alcohol, drugs, sedatives or food to help you relax? ☐
- Experience shakiness, trembling or cold hands? ☐
- Get sensitive to bright lights or loud noises? ☐
- Have problems finding the right words to say? ☐
- Find it hard to fall asleep? ☐

Total score ☐

Low acetylcholine levels

Do you:

- Have difficulty remembering people's names and/or
  birth dates? (multiply your score by 2) ☐
- Experience slow or confused thinking?
  (multiply your score by 2) ☐
- Have a poor memory or keep forgetting common facts?
  (multiply your score by 2) ☐

- Experience a dry mouth? ☐
- Struggle to find the right words before speaking? ☐
- Have difficulty visualising? ☐
- Experience despair and a lack of joy? ☐
- Have restless legs? ☐
- Crave or binge on fatty food? ☐
- Have poor dream recall? ☐

Total score ☐

Low dopamine levels

Do you:

- Have low energy, drive and/or enthusiasm?
  (multiply your score by 2) ☐
- Put on weight easily and/or rapidly?
  (multiply your score by 2) ☐
- Require excessive amounts of sleep and/or have
  difficulty getting out of bed in the morning?
  (multiply your score by 2) ☐
- Experience apathy or boredom or feel emotionally flat? ☐
- Have a reduced ability to feel pleasure? ☐
- Feel tired a lot of the time? ☐
- Experience repetitive, angry, guilty or self-critical thoughts? ☐
- Get chilled easily? ☐
- Have a poor attention span and/or difficulty concentrating? ☐
- Do you crave, binge on, or rely on, sugar, cocaine, nicotine
  and/or caffeine to give you a boost? ☐

Total score ☐

Nutritional imbalances

In this section you are going to identify which, if any, of the most common nutritional imbalances are preventing you from experiencing your emotional health potential. Although you're probably aware of most of the topics in this section, you may not have heard of methylation. It is a vital biological process that helps fine-tune your body chemistry. How well your body is performing this task is indicated by the level of a substance in the blood called homocysteine. Don't worry if you haven't had your level tested, other factors can indicate if sub-optimal methylation may be a problem for you.

Score the questionnaires as follows:

No = 0, Occasionally = 1, Yes = 2

If you answer 'Yes' to a question where you see an instruction in brackets, follow those instructions. Once you have added up your scores for each questionnaire, insert your totals in the score chart on page 138 or in your notebook or journal.

NUTRITIONAL IMBALANCE QUESTIONNAIRES

Dysglycemia (fluctuating blood-sugar levels)

Do you:

- Crave sweet foods or stimulants, such as caffeine or nicotine? (multiply your score by 2)

- Experience forgetfulness, poor memory or mental confusion, particularly after eating? (multiply your score by 2)

- Experience a drop in energy, mood or drowsiness after meals? (multiply your score by 2)

- Struggle with your weight despite watching what you eat?

- Experience forgetfulness, poor memory or mental confusion, particularly after eating?

- Store most of your body fat around your middle?

- Feel weak? □

- Experience frequent mood swings? □

- Have a tendency to night sweats or excessive sweating during the day? □

- Get excessively thirsty? □

Total score □

Sub-optimal methylation (related to B-vitamin deficiency)

Do you:

- Have a homocysteine level greater than 7 units (mmol/l)? (multiply your score by 6) □

- Have a personal history of heart disease, stroke, Alzheimer's disease or cancer? (multiply your score by 2) □

- Not take a multivitamin mineral or B-complex? (multiply your score by 2) □

- Eat fewer than five portions of fruits and vegetables a day? □

- Have a family history of heart disease, stroke, Alzheimer's disease or cancer? □

- Smoke cigarettes? □

- Have more than three alcoholic drinks a week? □

- Have a high intake of red meat and/or dairy? □

- Have a history of inflammatory bowel disease? □

- Have depression or a history of depression? □

Total score □

Zinc deficiency

Do you:

- Have an impairment of your ability to taste or smell? (multiply your score by 2) □

- Have eczema and/or acne? (multiply your score by 2) ☐
- Have white marks on more than two fingernails? (multiply your score by 2) ☐
- Drink hard water? ☐
- Take diuretics? ☐
- Sweat excessively? ☐
- Experience hair loss? ☐
- Have greasy skin? ☐
- Get repeated infections? ☐
- Have wounds that are healing poorly? ☐

Total score ☐

Magnesium deficiency

Do you:

- Experience muscle twitching or leg cramps? (multiply your score by 2) ☐
- Experience restless legs? (multiply your score by 2) ☐
- Experience difficulty in relaxing? (multiply your score by 2) ☐
- Have an irregular heart rhythm? ☐
- Have ADHD? ☐
- Experience anxiety, nervousness and/or irritability? ☐
- Have depression? ☐
- Get constipated? ☐
- Have a poor or deteriorating memory? ☐
- Have asthma? ☐

Total score ☐

Allergies and intolerances

In this section you are going to identify whether any allergies or food intolerances are preventing you from experiencing your emotional health potential.

No = 0, Occasionally = 1, Yes = 2

If you answer 'Yes' to a question where you see an instruction in brackets, follow those instructions. Once you have added up your scores for each questionnaire, insert your totals in the score chart on page 138 or in your notebook or journal.

QUESTIONNAIRE: Allergies and intolerances

Do you:

- Experience sudden, unexplained changes in mood, such as depression, anger, hyperactivity, irritability, depression and/or aggression? (multiply your score by 3)

- Find that fasting or skipping meals makes you more clear-headed and alert? (multiply your score by 2)

- Have dark circles under your eyes and/or facial puffiness? (multiply your score by 2)

- Have brain 'fog' or feelings of being 'spaced out'? (multiply your score by 2)

- Need to clear your nose/throat frequently and/or get a gritty feeling in your eyes? (multiply your score by 2)

- Get infections, and/or experience excess mucus or catarrh formation in the throat, nose, ear, lungs or sinuses?

- Have cravings for certain foods, such as chocolate, cheese or bread?

- Suffer from migraines, irritable bowel syndrome or regular headaches?

- Experience periods of clumsiness, poor concentration, inability to think clearly, blankness or momentary difficulty in finding the right word and/or poor comprehension? ☐

- Get abdominal bloating, pain and/or cramps? ☐

Total score ☐

Hormone imbalances

In this section you are going to identify which, if any, of the most common hormone imbalances is preventing you from experiencing your emotional health potential.

No = 0, Occasionally = 1, Yes = 2

If you answer 'Yes' to a question where you see an instruction in brackets, follow those instructions. Once you have added up your scores for each questionnaire, insert your totals in the score chart on page 138 or in your notebook or journal.

HORMONE IMBALANCE QUESTIONNAIRES

Adrenal fatigue

Do you:

- Feel stressed, restless, overwhelmed and/or exhausted? (multiply your score by 3) ☐

- Experience anxiety, nervousness, irritability, phobias or panic attacks? (multiply your score by 2) ☐

- Keep yourself going on sugar, caffeine and/or snacks? (multiply your score by 2) ☐

- Experience light-headedness on standing? ☐

- Feel more awake at night? ☐

- Crave salty foods, sugar or liquorice? ☐

- Have dark circles under your eyes or are your eyes sensitive to bright lights? □

- Spend the whole day rushing from one thing to another? □

- Suffer from interrupted sleep or insomnia? □

- Get absent-minded or feel that your short-term memory lets you down? □

Total score □

Hypothyroidism

Do you:

- Get easily chilled (especially hands and feet)? (multiply your score by 3) □

- Gain weight easily despite eating little/find it hard to lose excess weight? (multiply your score by 3) □

- Experience low energy levels or times when your energy levels suddenly drop? (multiply your score by 3) □

- Have a personal or family history of thyroid problems or autoimmune disorders (multiply your score by 3) □

- Experience a sore throat, a hoarse voice or problems swallowing? □

- Have a tendency to constipation and/or slow reflexes? □

- Have adult acne, dry skin or puffiness around the eyes? □

- Have dry hair or hair that falls out or loss of outer eyebrows? □

- Have brittle, thin, cracked or peeling nails? □

- Have depression and/or irritability? □

Total score □

Oestrogen/progesterone imbalance (women)

Do you:

- Experience premenstrual mood swings?
  (multiply your score by 2)

- Use or have you used birth-control pills or hormone
  medication?

- Experience irregular, lengthy or uncomfortable periods?
  (multiply your score by 2)

- Experience peri- or post-menopausal discomfort
  (such as hot flushes, weight gain, sweats or insomnia)?
  (multiply your score by 5)

- Have acne, excessive facial hair and/or have PCOS?
  (multiply your score by 5)

- Have a history of miscarriage or infertility?

- Have painful or lumpy breasts?

- Experience cyclical headaches or migraines?

- Gain weight easily or find it hard to lose weight?

  Total score

Testosterone imbalance (men)

Do you:

- Have any memory lapses, foggy thinking or periods
  of forgetfulness? (multiply your score by 3)

- Have a reduced sex drive? (multiply your score by 2)

- Experience problems getting a firm erection?
  (multiply your score by 2)

- Find that you are losing muscle mass and/or getting increased
  amounts of abdominal fat? (multiply your score by 2)

- Experience apathy and low energy levels? ☐

- Find that you are experiencing an increase in fatigue and deteriorating stamina? ☐

- Have enlargement of your breasts? ☐

- Experience any prostate problems, such as difficulty urinating or poor urine stream? ☐

- Have depression? ☐

- Have joint stiffness, aches or pains that aren't related to arthritis? ☐

Total score ☐

Dysbiosis

In this section you are going to identify whether dysbiosis (a state of imbalance in which the normal healthy population of beneficial bacteria in the intestines has been disrupted) is preventing you from experiencing your emotional health potential.

No = 0, Occasionally = 1, Yes = 2

If you answer 'Yes' to a question where you see an instruction in brackets, follow those instructions. Once you have added up your scores, insert your total in the score chart on page 138 or in your notebook or journal.

QUESTIONNAIRE: Dysbiosis

Do you:

- Have a diagnosis of yeast, candida and/or parasites? (multiply your score by 6) ☐

- Crave alcohol, sugar and/or bread? (multiply your score by 2) ☐

- Get recurring digestive problems, such as abdominal bloating, excessive wind, heartburn, diarrhoea or constipation? (multiply your score by 2) ☐

- Get yeast infections, such as thrush? (multiply your score by 2) ☐

- Experience foggy-headedness or unexplained migraines? ☐

- Experience unexplained tiredness, poor concentration and/or depression? ☐

- Have a history of using steroids or birth-control pills for more than one year? ☐

- Have chronic fungus on your nails, skin or athlete's foot? ☐

- Have stools of an unusual colour, shape or consistency? ☐

- Have any food allergies or intolerances? ☐

Total score ☐

Your scores

Having completed the questionnaires, the next step is to transfer your scores to the chart below or, if you prefer, to a notebook or journal. A score of 12 or more on any questionnaire suggests that you would benefit from the advice I provide in the next section. If you score over 12 in more than one, start with the highest-scoring one first; alternatively work with an experienced integrative medical doctor or a doctor who specialises in ecological medicine (see Resources, page 276).

Imbalance	Your score
Neurotransmitter imbalances	
Serotonin	☐
GABA	☐
Acetylcholine	☐
Dopamine	☐

Nutritional imbalances

Dysglycemia ☐

Methylation (B vitamins) ☐

Zinc ☐

Magnesium ☐

Allergies and food intolerances ☐

Hormone imbalances

Adrenal ☐

Thyroid ☐

Sex hormones ☐

Dysbiosis ☐

Having completed the questionnaires and identified which of the bio-chemical and physical imbalances are most relevant to you, the next step is to work through the suggestions that address them. In each section, under 'Address the underlying causes', you will find sugges-tions on the appropriate pillars for that particular imbalance. As I have said previously, if you feel overwhelmed or have more than three imbalances, I'd highly recommend that you work with an integrative medicine doctor or nutritional therapist.

OTHER FACTORS THAT CAN CAUSE IMBALANCES

In addition to the factors already discussed there is a variety of other factors that can contribute to mood problems and which I consider in most of my patients. In a nutshell, they are as follows:

- Heavy metal toxins, such as mercury, cadmium, aluminium, copper and lead: these are increasingly being recognised as being contributors (albeit relatively rare) to a wide variety of mental and emotional health problems and symptoms.[55] (See the healthy environment section in Pillar Four, page 121, for more information on mercury toxicity.)

- Chemical toxicity and contaminants from food, air, water and the products we use and are exposed to: these can, in particular, interfere with the brain's neurotransmitters and block the action of a variety of important vitamins.[56] (See the healthy environment section in Pillar Four, page 121, for more information.)

- Low-grade inflammation over the body: this is increasingly being recognised as one of the major common contributors to over a hundred different diseases including autism, Alzheimer's, depression, heart disease and cancer.[57]

- Medications: these can be a cause of or contributor to a disturbed mood or mental-health problems. Look up the side effects of any medications you are on and discuss these with the doctor who prescribed them.

- Disease and illness: any infectious, inflammatory or chronic health issues can contribute to mood problems. This is because of the disease processes' effects on the body's biochemistry and because illnesses often make it more challenging for us to meet our physical and emotional needs in a balanced and moderate way.

- Structural problems relating to spinal misalignment and distortion of the skull: if you have any back/neck problems or have experienced physical trauma you might want to consider having an osteopathic, cranial osteopathic or chiropractic assessment to see if misalignment of your vertebrae (the building blocks of the spine) is negatively impacting on your mental health and mood.[58]

My book The Mind–Body Bible covers these factors in more depth. If you suspect that any of the above applies to you, or if your have mood problems that don't resolve with the suggestions in this book, you should consider working with a medical doctor who specialises in integrative medicine or ecological medicine (which examines allergy, environmental and nutritional factors).

Neurotransmitter imbalances

Your emotional health and happiness are intimately connected to your neurotransmitter levels. As I pointed out previously, neurotransmitters are the chemical messengers of the nervous system that relay information around and between the brain and body, enabling the different parts of the body and brain to talk to one another.

The human brain has roughly 10 trillion nerve cells (neurons) that communicate with one another through synaptic connections. When activated, a nerve cell will release neurotransmitters into the synaptic cleft, the space between it and the adjacent nerve cell. They then move across this space and dock on to the next cell's receptor sites and, depending on the nature of the docked neurotransmitter, this will trigger a variety of chemical reactions. The majority of the original neurotransmitters will then be taken back up into the original cell. A whole class of antidepressants called SSRIs work by preventing this from happening.

The four main neurotransmitters

While there are many important neurotransmitters, four of the most important for emotional health and happiness are the two so-called inhibitory neurotransmitters serotonin and GABA and two excitatory neurotransmitters acetylcholine and dopamine (and its derivatives adrenaline and noradrenaline). The excitatory ones, as their name suggests, are designed to make you focused, aroused, energised, stimulated and able to learn and remember. The inhibitory ones take you in the other direction; their job is to make you feel calm, relaxed, peaceful and content. The key, from an emotional health perspective, is to ensure that all of these are kept in balance.

Serotonin

Serotonin is produced from the amino acid tryptophan and plays a major role in emotional and mental health. When balanced, it creates feelings of calm and contentment. In addition to influencing mood, it is also linked to appetite, pain perception, body temperature, sexual desire, regulation of sleep and blood pressure. Low serotonin levels might be associated with (but not necessarily the cause of) depression, food cravings, anxiety, insomnia, eating disorders, anger, OCD, PMS and alcohol/drug abuse.[59]

If you scored 12 or more on the low serotonin questionnaire, you'd benefit from taking the following steps.

Address the underlying causes of low serotonin levels

The underlying causes of, and contributors to, your low serotonin levels may be:

- Poor diet (see below and Pillar Four)
- Stress (Pillar Six)
- Nutritional deficiencies (Pillars Four and Five)
- Hormone imbalance (Pillar Five)
- Excessive intake of alcohol and caffeine; smoking (addictions, Pillars Four and Six)
- Dysbiosis (Pillar Five)
- Lack of physical activity (Pillar Four)
- Toxicity (Pillar Five)
- Poor emotional management (Pillars One and Two)
- Not meeting your emotional needs (Pillar Three)

Make dietary adjustments

- Increase your intake of foods that are high in tryptophan, the precursor amino acid for serotonin: grass-fed meat, eggs, chicken, turkey, nuts, seeds and bananas.

- Take a multivitamin–mineral–antioxidant, vitamin C with bioflavonoids and fish oil/flaxseed oil (see Pillar Four) and consider taking 5-HTP or St John's Wort. The mood-stabilising effects of 5-HTP (produced commercially by extraction from the seeds of the

African plant, *Griffonia simplicifolia*) are believed to result from its ability to increase the production of serotonin levels in the brain.[60] The recommended dose is between 50mg and 150mg, twice a day. Take with a non-protein snack, such as a small piece of fruit or oatcake as this helps to improve its effectiveness. In my experience, and as long as they are addressing Pillars One to Four, however, most people do not need to take 5-HTP for more than six months.

Note: if you take 5-HTP and start developing irritability, headaches, vivid dreams, nausea or excessive sleepiness, reduce your evening and/or mid-afternoon dose by 50mg, until symptoms disappear. Do not take 5-HTP if you have heart disease, are pregnant, breast-feeding or are on antidepressants. In addition, 5-HTP may exacerbate asthma – if this occurs you should stop taking it. You should also start with a low dose of 5-HTP if you have a pre-existing intestinal problem, such as ulcers or IBS, as the likelihood of experiencing side effects may be greater.

- As an alternative to 5-HTP or if you have not had a positive response with 5-HTP, you might want to consider using St John's Wort. This is the best researched of all of the alternative natural antidepressants. In Germany, more than 50 per cent of patients with mild/moderate depression, anxiety and sleep disorders are treated with St John's Wort.[61] The recommended dose is 300mg, three times daily, standardised to 0.9 mg hypericin.

Note: you shouldn't take St John's Wort if you are taking the oestrogen contraceptive pill, antidepressants, warfarin, digoxin, MAO inhibitors or if you have a diagnosis of manic depression.

GABA

GABA is produced from the amino acid glutamine with the help of vitamin B_6. When balanced, it helps you to keep relaxed and calm. It also controls muscle activity and is important for healthy vision. Low GABA levels might be associated with (but not necessarily the cause of) anxiety, panic attacks, irritability, schizophrenia, insomnia and addictions.[62]

If you scored 12 or more on the low GABA questionnaire, you'd benefit from taking the following steps.

Address the underlying causes of low GABA levels

The underlying causes of, and contributors to, your low GABA levels might be:

- Poor diet (see below and Pillar Four)

- Stress (Pillar Six)

- Nutritional deficiencies (Pillars Four and Five)

- Hormone imbalance (Pillar Five)

- Excessive intake of alcohol and caffeine, smoking (addictions, Pillars Four and Six)

- Dysbiosis (Pillar Five)

- Lack of physical activity (Pillar Four)

- Toxicity (Pillar Five)

- Poor emotional management (Pillars One and Two)

- Not meeting your emotional needs (Pillar Three)

Make dietary adjustments

- Increase your intake of foods that are high in glutamic acid/glutamate, the precursor amino acids for glutamine and GABA: wholegrains, nuts (walnuts, almonds), oats, spinach, broccoli, bananas, organ meats and brown rice.

- In addition to taking a multivitamin–mineral–antioxidant, vitamin C with bioflavonoids and fish oil/flaxseed oil (see Pillar Four), consider taking L-theanine. The amino acid L-theanine, a green tea extract, can help to create a sense of relaxation within approximately thirty to forty minutes of ingestion, by increasing levels of GABA.[63] The relaxation effect lasts for up to eight hours. The recommended dose is 50–200mg (depending on severity of problem), twice a day and it can also be taken in combination with other relaxation-inducing ingredients, such as magnesium, passion flower, lemon balm and B vitamins (see Resources, page 283).

Acetylcholine

Acetylcholine is produced from the B vitamin choline and a molecule called acetyl. It is responsible for stimulating many of the body's muscles, including those of the gastrointestinal system and for causing glands to release hormones. It is also related to learning and memory. Low acetylcholine levels might be associated with (but not necessarily the cause of) poor memory function and Alzheimer's disease.[64]

If you scored 12 or more on the low acetylcholine questionnaire, you'd benefit from taking the following steps.

Address the underlying causes of low acetylcholine levels

The underlying causes of and contributors to your low acetylcholine levels might be:

- Poor diet (see below and Pillar Four)

- Stress (Pillar Six)

- Nutritional deficiencies (Pillars Four and Five)

- Hormone imbalance (Pillar Five)

- Excessive intake of alcohol and caffeine, smoking (addictions, Pillars Four and Six)

- Dysbiosis (Pillar Five)

- Lack of physical activity (Pillar Four)

- Toxicity (Pillar Five)

- Poor emotional management (Pillars One and Two)

- Not meeting your emotional needs (Pillar Three)

Make dietary adjustments

- Increase your intake of foods that are high in choline, the precursor to acetylcholine: egg yolk, organ meats, beef, tofu, soya beans, almonds, butter, cabbage, cauliflower, tomatoes, bananas, lentils and oats.

- In addition to taking a multivitamin–mineral–antioxidant, vitamin C with bioflavonoids and fish oil/flaxseed oil (see Pillar Four), you should also consider taking lecithin. Also called phosphatidyl choline (PC), it is a phospholipid that is essential to mood, memory, clear thinking and mental performance.[65] It provides the B vitamin choline which gets converted in the body to acetylcholine. The recommended daily dose is a tablespoon of lecithin granules (about 5g) or a heaped teaspoon of high PC sprinkled over your cereal or into your yoghurt every day.[66] If you are eating choline-rich foods, you don't need as much.

Note: reduce your dose if you experience abdominal discomfort, diarrhoea or nausea.

Dopamine

Dopamine is produced by the two amino acids tyrosine and l-phenylalanine, and when released by the brain it produces feelings of pleasure. It also helps with motivation, drive, concentration and memory. Low dopamine levels might be associated with (but not necessarily the cause of) low energy, depression, addictions, ADHD and Parkinson's disease.[67] Dopamine is converted in the body to noradrenaline and adrenaline, two other powerful neurotransmitters. Both of these have a strong influence on your ability to hold your attention, focus and levels of arousal.

If you scored 12 or more on the low dopamine questionnaire, you'd benefit from taking the following steps.

Address the underlying causes of low dopamine levels

The underlying causes of and contributors to your low dopamine levels might be:

- Poor diet (see below and Pillar Four)

- Stress (Pillar Six)

- Nutritional deficiencies (Pillars Four and Five)

- Hormone imbalance (Pillar Five)

- Excessive intake of alcohol and caffeine, smoking (addictions, Pillars Four and Six)

- Dysbiosis (Pillar Five)

- Lack of physical activity (Pillar Four)

- Toxicity (Pillar Five)

- Poor emotional management (Pillars One and Two)

- Not meeting your emotional needs (Pillar Three)

Make dietary adjustments

- Increase your intake of foods that are high in L-tyrosine, the precursor amino acid to dopamine, noradrenaline and adrenaline: grass-fed meat, eggs, chicken and fish.

- In addition to taking a multivitamin–mineral–antioxidant, vitamin C with bioflavonoids and fish oil/flaxseed oil (see Pillar Four), consider taking L-tyrosine and/or L-phenylalanine. The recommended dose is between 500mg and 1000mg, three times a day (before breakfast, mid-morning and mid-afternoon). If you start to feel jittery, tense, nervous or have headaches, raised blood pressure or problems getting to sleep, reduce your total daily dose and/or omit the afternoon one (if insomnia is the problem). In my experience, and as long as they are addressing Pillars One to Four, most people do not need to take L-tyrosine for more than one or two months.

  Note: do not take L-tyrosine unless medically advised to do so if you have a history of manic depression, phenylketonuria, hashimoto's thyroiditis, hyperthyroidism, migraines, high blood pressure or melanoma.

- If L-tyrosine isn't helping you, you could consider adding in, or using as an alternative, another amino acid called L-phenylalanine. This is converted in the liver to L-tyrosine, then dopamine, noradrenaline and adrenaline.[68] The recommended dose of L-phenylalanine is between 500mg and 1000mg, three times a day (before breakfast, mid-morning and mid-afternoon). If you are combining it with L-tyrosine you should use much lower dosages and do so under the supervision of a medical doctor or nutritional therapist.

Note: do not take phenylalanine supplements if you have phenylketonuria (PKU) or schizophrenia, or you are pregnant or breastfeeding. Also, L-phenylalanine, like L-tyrosine may cause symptoms of anxiety, jitteriness and hyperactivity; you should reduce your dose or stop taking them if you experience any of these.

Nutritional imbalances

Nutritional imbalances are a common contributor to mood and mental health problems. If you haven't already done so, I would encourage you to read the 'Optimise your nutrition' section in Pillar Four, then follow the specific recommendations below.

The main nutritional imbalances

Blood-sugar imbalance (dysglycemia)

Dysglycemia, or fluctuating blood-sugar levels, is one of the most common contributors to tiredness, mood swings, irritability and poor concentration that I see in my patients.[69] I have covered in some detail already how to go about balancing your blood sugar using diet and supplements in Pillar Four.

If you scored 12 or more on the dysglycemia questionnaire, you'd benefit from taking the following steps.

See your doctor

Consider asking your doctor to do a blood test to measure your level of glycosylated haemoglobin; this will tell you whether your blood-sugar level has been swinging too high or low. Your GP should also check for diabetes, if that is suspected.

Address the underlying causes of dysglycemia

The underlying causes of and contributors to your dysglycemia might be:

- Poor diet (see below and Pillar Four)

- Stress (Pillar Six)

- Nutritional deficiencies (Pillars Four and Five)

- Hormone imbalance (Pillar Five)

- Excessive intake of alcohol and caffeine, smoking (addictions, Pillars Four and Six)

- Sleep deprivation (Pillar Four)

- Dysbiosis (Pillar Five)

- Lack of physical activity (Pillar Four)

- Toxicity (Pillar Five)

- Poor emotional management (Pillars One and Two)

- Not meeting your emotional needs (Pillar Three)

Make dietary adjustments

- In addition to taking a multivitamin–mineral–antioxidant, vitamin C with bioflavonoids and fish oil[70] – 3000mg a day (see Pillar Four) or flaxseed oil, you should also consider taking chromium polynicotinate (400–1000mcg a day, depending on severity) or chromium with GTF (1 to 3 tablets a day). GTF stands for glucose tolerance factor and refers to a special type of chromium, first isolated from brewer's yeast, which is a complex of chromium, vitamin B_3 and three amino acids. This is the form of chromium that works closely with insulin in facilitating the uptake of glucose into cells.[71]

- Other supplements to take include: alpha-lipoic acid (100mg three times a day) – this is an antioxidant that can improve insulin resistance and increase glucose uptake into muscle cells;[72] co-enzyme Q10 (30mg a day) – this may help to improve the function of insulin-producing cells in the pancreas, as well as lower blood pressure and raise HDL cholesterol levels;[73] and glutamine (a heaped teaspoon in water, sipped throughout the day) – this is an amino acid that can greatly aid blood sugar and appetite control (it helps prevent hypoglycaemia because it is easily converted to glucose when blood sugar dips, also helping to prevent cravings and overeating).

- The key to correcting dysglycemia from a dietary perspective is to eat regularly (three meals and two snacks – one mid-morning and one mid-afternoon), eat protein with each meal and snack and limit foods that are known to interfere negatively with blood-sugar imbalance (such as, white bread, sugary breakfast cereals, white rice, potatoes, crisps, overcooked white pasta, sugar-rich cakes, pastries and sweets). See Optimise Your Nutrition in Pillar Four, page 93, for more information on healthy eating.

Sub-optimal methylation

Methylation is one of the most important factors in keeping your hormones and neurotransmitters in balance. At the most basic level, methylation is the process by which a carbon-containing molecule called a methyl group is passed on to another molecule. This transaction allows the smooth running and functioning of over a hundred different processes in the body, including switching on and off the expression of certain genes, building proteins and influencing the levels and activity of the mood-influencing neurotransmitters. The latter is particularly relevant to your emotional and mental health. When the process of methylation isn't working effectively, due to either a poor diet (in particular one low in B vitamins), stress, hormone imbalances or a genetic propensity to under-methylation, it leads to low levels of serotonin, noradrenaline and dopamine, which, in turn, increase the likelihood of you developing depression.

If you scored 12 or more on the methylation questionnaire, you'd benefit from taking the following steps.

Take a homocysteine test

This test measures the level of the amino acid homocysteine, which is often raised if you have a faulty methylation system due to the causes mentioned above and/or a genetically inherited mutation in the gene that controls the conversion of homocysteine into a substance called SAMe (which is needed for optimal mental health). Raised homocysteine levels have been linked to a variety of health problems including schizophrenia, Alzheimer's disease, depression and diabetes.[74] A healthy homocysteine level is under 7 mmol/l. (See Resources, page 283 for further details.)

Address the underlying causes of sub-optimal methylation

The underlying causes of and contributors to sub-optimal methylation might be:

- Poor diet (see below and Pillar Four)

- Stress (Pillar Six)

- Hormone imbalance (Pillar Five)

- Excessive intake of alcohol and caffeine, smoking (addictions, Pillars Four and Six)

- Dysbiosis (Pillar Five)

- Lack of physical activity (Pillar Four)

- Toxicity (Pillar Five)

- Poor emotional management (Pillars One and Two)

Make dietary adjustments

- Increase your intake of foods that are high in B vitamins, such as nuts, seeds, vegetables and beans.

- Consider taking the vitamins B_2, B_6, B_{12} and folate, all of which help to activate the enzymes that convert homocysteine into SAMe and the antioxidant glutathione. The best way to take these B vitamins is as part of a vitamin B complex or high-potency multivitamin–mineral. The optimum dose – though this will depend on you and your homocysteine level – is in the region of: 25–100mg) for B_2, 25–100mg for B_6, 10–1000mcg for B_{12} and 400–1000mcg for folic acid.

- In addition to the B vitamins, I recommend taking TMG (trimethyl glycine), which can help to lower homocysteine levels. You should take between 500mg and 3000mg a day, depending on your levels, until optimum levels are achieved.

- You should also take zinc at a dose of between 5mg and 15mg a day; it works with vitamin B_6 to promote the re-methylation of homocysteine.

Zinc

Zinc is an essential mineral that is necessary for the functioning of many of the body's enzymes, as well as the synthesis of DNA and protein. It's also important for a healthily functioning immune system, taste, blood clotting, sperm production, thyroid function and testosterone production. Deficiencies of zinc might be associated with (but not necessarily the cause of) a variety of mental-health issues including eating disorders, poor memory, PMS, lack of motivation, depression and loss of appetite.[75]

If you scored 12 or more on the zinc questionnaire, you'd benefit from taking the following steps.

Take a mineral test

I recommend using the mineral test kit I mentioned briefly in the supplements section (see page 110) to confirm a zinc deficiency.

Address the underlying causes of low zinc levels

The underlying causes of and contributors to your low zinc levels might be:

- Poor diet (see below and Pillar Four)

- High copper levels

- High intake of calcium

- Dysbiosis (Pillar Five)

- Stress (Pillar Six)

- Excessive intake of alcohol (Pillars Four and Six)

- Pregnancy or breastfeeding

- Chronic illness

Make dietary adjustments

- Increase your intake of zinc-rich foods: oysters, shellfish, wheat germ, wheat bran, nuts (pine, pecan and cashew), seeds (pumpkin and sesame), liver, mushrooms, fish, eggs, avocados, olives, tomatoes, vegetables (peas, spinach, sweet potatoes, cauliflower, onions, artichoke and cucumber), and fruit (peaches, kiwi, blackberries, strawberries and bananas).

- When replacing zinc I recommend using a zinc product that can be taken sublingually (under the tongue) or as a liquid (see Resources, page 283 for more information). Because zinc is an antagonist to iron, manganese and copper, if you are taking more than 20mg a day, you should ensure that you are also supplementing these three as well. A high-potency multivitamin–mineral will usually supply these.

Note: don't take more than 40mg of zinc a day unless under the supervision of a medical doctor or nutritional therapist. If you do take a high dose, you should reduce it to no more than 10mg a day after one to two months. Repeating the zinc taste test will let you know when to cut back.

Magnesium

Magnesium is another essential mineral that is essential for bone health, improving insulin sensitivity, heart-rhythm stabilisation, controlling blood pressure and regulating over 300 enzymes. Deficiencies of magnesium might be associated with (but not necessarily the cause of) a variety of mental-health issues including anxiety, insomnia, tension, ADHD, irritability and PMS.[76]

If you scored 12 or more on the magnesium questionnaire, you'd benefit from taking the following steps.

Take a mineral test

I recommend using the mineral test kit I mentioned briefly in the supplements section (page 110) to confirm a magnesium deficiency.

Address the underlying causes of low magnesium levels

The underlying causes of and contributors to your low magnesium levels might be:

- Poor diet (see below and Pillar Four)
- High intake of calcium
- Dysbiosis (Pillar Five)
- Stress (Pillar Six)
- Excessive intake of alcohol (Pillars Four and Six)
- Excessive or prolonged diarrhoea or vomiting
- Taking diuretics (tablets that help to treat high blood pressure and oedema)

Make dietary adjustments

- Increase your intake of magnesium-rich foods: spinach, Swiss chard, kale, broccoli, mustard greens, pumpkin seeds, celery, cucumber, green beans and seeds (sesame, sunflower and flax).
- When taking magnesium supplements, you should consider taking between 400mg and 600mg of magnesium citrate, ascorbate, aspartate or glycinate, either in tablet or liquid form.

  Note: the most common side effect of magnesium supplements is diarrhoea; others include nausea and abdominal cramping. If these occur, reduce your dose and take with food as this reduces the likelihood of side effects.

  Also, avoid magnesium supplements altogether if you have kidney failure or myasthenia gravis.

For recommended further reading on all of the above, see Resources, page 290.

Allergies and intolerances

If you experience mood swings, foggy thinking or problems with keeping your focus, you are probably suffering the consequences of allergies on the brain.[77] In fact, allergies, particularly to food, are increasingly being recognised as a significant and commonly undiagnosed contributor to our emotional and mental health. Some studies, for example, have found a speculative link between gluten (the protein found in wheat, barley, rye, spelt and oats) and schizophrenia, depression, anxiety, psychosis and autism. The way this works is that, firstly, the body reacts to it and triggers an inflammatory response in the brain. Next, food proteins, called peptides from gluten and casein (milk), are known to disrupt normal neurotransmitter function in the brain. Finally, food-allergy reactions are known to stimulate the production of an excitatory neurotransmitter called glutamate, which can lead to damage and inflammation of certain brain cells.

A common problem

In this section I am going to concentrate on food allergies and intolerances because these are the ones I most commonly see in clinical practice. Sensitivity to food additives, artificial flavourings, dyes and preservatives can also be a problem for people who get rapid mood swings. For this reason, and especially if you have multiple allergy symptoms, I recommend you consult with an allergy specialist or doctor specialising in ecological or environmental medicine. (See Resources, page 276, for more information.)

Food intolerances

Food intolerance is a term that is used to describe a range of detrimental responses to a specific food or food ingredient. It can include allergic reactions which involve the immune system (as in a peanut allergy or coeliac disease); reactions resulting from enzyme deficiencies (such as lactose intolerance, which affects 70 per cent of the world's population, but far fewer people of North European descent – about 2 per cent); sensitivities to certain types of food (such as yeast in people with candida); or pharmacological reactions (such as caffeine or sugar sensitivity). The most common food intolerances are to cow's milk and cheese, wheat, gluten (found in oats, wheat, rye and barley), corn, beef, yeast, eggs, garlic, nuts, seeds, kiwi and soya.

If you scored 12 or more on the allergies and intolerances questionnaire, you'd benefit from taking the following steps.

Confirm your diagnosis

There are a couple of ways in which to do this. You can do what's called an elimination diet, in which you remove suspect foods (such as wheat and dairy) for a few weeks, then cautiously reintroduce one food group every fourth day to see if the symptoms come back. Most people, however, find this too complicated. Another option is to go for a food allergen cellular test which measures levels of inflammatory chemicals released from white blood cells when they are exposed to various food allergens. (See Resources, page 282.)

If you get a positive test result, you should ideally avoid or limit consumption of the intolerance-evoking foods for at least three months and, while doing so, start addressing any underlying causes/contributors and take the supplements recommended below.

Address the underlying causes of food intolerance

The underlying causes of, and contributors to, your food intolerances might be:

- Leaky gut syndrome (in which the spaces in between the cells that line the intestines become irritated, inflamed and allow undigested food to enter the bloodstream)

- Poor diet (Pillar Four)

- Nutritional imbalances (Pillars Four and Five)

- Stress (Pillar Six)

- Non-steroidal anti-inflammatories or steroids

- Excessive intake of alcohol and caffeine, smoking (addictions, Pillars Four and Six)

- Inflammatory bowel disease, gut infection and dysbiosis (Pillar Five)

- Health problems, such as constipation and any inflammatory disease

Take dietary supplements

In addition to taking a multivitamin–mineral–antioxidant, vitamin C with bioflavonoids and fish oil – 1000–3000mg (as outlined in Pillar Four) or flaxseed oil (one to two tablespoons or capsules), you should also consider taking the following:

- L-glutamine (5g, once to three times daily) – this is an amino acid powder that can help to repair the lining of the small intestine (leaky gut); take for a minimum of one month.

- Butyric acid (1200mg a day) – this feeds the cells of the intestinal lining and is essential in maintaining the integrity of the gastrointestinal wall.

- A comprehensive digestive enzyme formula – this should be taken with each main meal if you get bloating or wind after eating and/or have undigested food in your stool. Take for one month (dose according to label) and then review.

- Acidophilus probiotic – this supports healthy gut and immune function by ensuring that there are sufficient numbers of 'friendly' bacteria in the gut. Take for a minimum of six months (dose according to label).

- Betaine hydrochloride (dose according to label) – this can help to improve stomach acid levels.

- Aloe vera – this plant extract contains a number of biologically active ingredients which are known to be anti-inflammatory, anti-bacterial and pro-healing for the gut and body. Take for one month (dose according to label).

Hormone imbalances

Hormone imbalances are a common contributor to mood problems (due to stress, poor diet, toxicity and not meeting physical/emotional needs) and should always be considered and addressed if present. In this section, I am going to cover those that I see most commonly in my patients.

Adrenal fatigue

If you are tired on waking up in the morning, chronically stressed out or suffer from any long-standing health problem, then you might be experiencing adrenal fatigue. The adrenals are two small pyramid-shaped glands sitting on top of your kidneys. Despite their small size, they are vitally important to your health and well-being – they help your body respond to stress, maintain the body's energy, regulate the immune system and keep your blood sugar, fluid levels and blood pressure within a healthy range. Healthy adrenal glands secrete very precise amounts of steroid hormones. However, too much ongoing physical, emotional, environmental and/or psychological stress can cause an imbalance in the function of the adrenals, and the result is adrenal fatigue, also known as adrenal burnout syndrome. This is a common condition that arises when the adrenal glands are no longer able to meet the demands placed upon them.

If you scored 12 or more on the adrenal fatigue questionnaire, you'd benefit from taking the following steps.

Take an adrenal stress index (ASI) saliva test

This test measures the level of two adrenal hormones – DHEA and cortisol – and provides a useful indicator of the severity of any adrenal fatigue. (See Resources, page 282 for details of supplier.)

Address the underlying causes of adrenal fatigue

The underlying causes of and contributors to your adrenal fatigue might be:

- Poor diet (Pillar Four)

- Stress (Pillar Six)

- Nutritional deficiencies (Pillars Four and Five)

- Hormone imbalance (Pillar Five)

- Excessive intake of alcohol and caffeine, smoking (addictions, Pillars Four and Six)

- Sleep deprivation (Pillar Four)

- Dysbiosis (Pillar Five)

- Lack of physical activity (Pillar Four)

- Toxicity (Pillar Five)

- Poor emotional management (Pillars One and Two)

- Not meeting your emotional needs (Pillar Three)

- Allergies (Pillar Five)

- Hypothyroidism (Pillar Five)

- Electropollution (Pillar Four)

- Depression and anxiety (Pillar Six)

- Dysglycemia (Pillars Four and Five)

Take dietary supplements

In addition to taking a multivitamin–mineral–antioxidant, vitamin C with bioflavonoids and fish oil/flaxseed oil (see Pillar Four), you should also consider taking the following:

- Pantothenic acid (500–600 mg a day) – this is also known as vitamin B_5 and is the most important 'anti-stress' B vitamin

- Magnesium (400–800mg a day) – this helps to relieve stress, tension and to support adrenal hormone manufacture

To these, I would also add one of the following adaptogenic herbs (these help the body to restore balance, fight fatigue and boost energy levels):

- Rhodiola (also called arctic root) – this works on an area of the brain called the hypothalamus to increase resistance to toxins and stress. It also helps to boost stamina and endurance, as well as increasing levels of the neurotransmitters, serotonin and dopamine.[78]

- Ashwagandha (also called Indian ginseng) – this works more as a nerve tonic. It balances the nervous system and the musculoskeletal system, enabling the body to relax and sleep.[79]

- Ginseng – this is another adaptogen that has been used for thousands of years in traditional Chinese medicine as a tonic to help the body reach its full potential for health. There are a few different types of ginseng, but those must useful for helping to recharge the adrenals are Siberian[80], Korean and American ginseng.[81]

- If your adrenal fatigue is severe, you might also benefit from taking liquorice extract and possibly the hormones pregnenolone and/or 7-keto DHEA. However, this should only be done under the supervision of a medical doctor or nutritional therapist.

Hypothyroidism

An estimated one in ten people suffers from hypothyroidism, an underactive thyroid gland – and the majority don't know it.[82] Women are at the greatest risk, developing thyroid problems seven times more often than men, with the risk increasing with age and for those with a family history of thyroid problems. Left untreated, thyroid imbalances can leave people at risk of heart disease, infertility and osteoporosis.

Your thyroid is a butterfly-shaped gland that curves around your windpipe. The cells that make up the thyroid gland combine the mineral iodine with the amino-acid L-tyrosine to create two hormones – thyroxine (T4) and the biologically more active triiodothyronine (T3). Once released by the thyroid gland, these hormones travel throughout the body and regulate the enzymes involved in controlling the rate at which bodily functions occur. If thyroid hormone levels are high, everything speeds up – your heart quickens, you lose weight and you find it hard to switch off. If thyroid hormone levels are too low, everything slows down – you become constipated, tired and mentally slow.

Hypothyroidism tends to occur when the thyroid gland fails to make sufficient thyroid hormone to meet the body's demand. This gives the classic symptoms of low energy, low temperature, extreme tiredness, intolerance to cold weather, mental drowsiness, weight gain, depression, low libido, thinning hair and constipation.

WHAT CAUSES HYPOTHYROIDISM?

Many different factors can affect thyroid function. One of the most common is an auto-immune disease, namely Ord's disease and Hashimoto's disease, in which antibodies are produced and directed towards the thyroid gland. This might be triggered by a viral infection or be due to a genetic vulnerability. Other known causes include chronic stress; adrenal fatigue; mineral deficiencies, such as iodine, selenium and zinc; a deficiency of tyrosine (the amino acid precursor to T4); toxicity and mercury intoxication; a tumour of the pituitary gland; certain medications, such as lithium (used to treat some kinds of depression), amiodarone (used to treat abnormal heart rhythms) and interferon (used to treat hepatitis); and thyroid surgery.

If you scored 12 or more on the hypothyroidism questionnaire, you'd benefit from taking the following steps.

Get a blood test

You will need to get a blood test to confirm the diagnosis; your GP should be able to arrange this.

Address the underlying causes of hypothyroidism

The underlying causes of and contributors to your hypothyroidism might be:

- Poor diet (see below and Pillar Four)

- Stress (Pillar Six)

- Nutritional deficiencies (Pillars Four and Five)

- Hormone imbalances (Pillar Five)

- Excessive intake of alcohol and caffeine, smoking (addictions, Pillars Four and Six)

- Sleep deprivation (Pillar Four)

- Dysbiosis (Pillar Five)

- Lack of physical activity (Pillar Four)

- Toxicity (Pillar Five)

- Poor emotional management (Pillars One and Two)

- Not meeting your emotional needs (Pillar Three)

- Allergies (Pillar Five)

- Adrenal fatigue (Pillar Five)

- Electropollution (Pillar Four)

- Depression and anxiety (Pillar Six)

- Dysglycemia (Pillars Four and Five)

Thyroid replacement therapy

Most people with hypothyroidism, and certainly those with autoimmune thyroid disease, will require treatment with thyroid replacement therapy. This usually consists of synthetic T4 (synthroid), either with or without synthetic T3 (usually called Cytomel). An alternative preferred by some doctors is armour thyroid, a prescription medication that contains desiccated thyroid derived from the thyroid gland of the pig. Some people reportedly do better on this, possibly because it contains a mix of T4 and T3 (see Resources, page 284, for more information).

Make dietary adjustments

- Limit your intake of goitrogens – foods that interfere with the release of thyroid hormone and with the conversion of T4 to T3.

These include soya, walnuts, peanuts, almonds, millet, pine nuts, vegetables from the brassica family (such as cabbage and turnips), mustard and apples. However, when these are cooked, the compounds that cause thyroid imbalance are inactivated. Foods that help stimulate thyroid hormone production and the conversion of T4 to T3 include egg yolk, seaweeds (kelp and dulse), mushrooms, garlic, seafood and wheatgerm. Coconut oil is also thyroid-stimulating and should be used in cooking.

- In addition to taking a multivitamin–mineral–antioxidant, vitamin C with bioflavonoids and fish oil/flaxseed oil (see Pillar Four), you should also consider taking L-tyrosine (500mg twice a day). This is an energising amino acid that's used in the synthesis of thyroid hormones. Also, kelp (take according to manufacturer's instructions) is a potent source of iodine and useful if iodine deficiency is suspected.[83]

Note: do not take kelp if you have Ord's or Hashimoto's thyroiditis, as it can aggravate the condition.

Oestrogen/progesterone imbalance (women)

The sex hormones oestrogen, progesterone and testosterone have a direct effect on your brain, mind, mood and memory.

Oestrogen enhances the production of serotonin, while increasing the number of serotonin receptor sites in parts of the brain. Too little oestrogen is associated with depression, loss of libido, high blood pressure, weight gain, hot flushes, excessive sweating and a dry vagina. Too much causes over-excitability of the brain which may contribute to anxiety and insomnia, as well as an increased risk of cervical, uterine and breast cancer.

Progesterone, on the other hand, has a calming effect on the brain by stimulating GABA receptors. It can also help to improve focus and concentration. Too little progesterone is associated with anxiety, depression, insomnia, mood swings and irritability, as well as fibroids, weight gain, excessive menstruation and osteoporosis. Too much progesterone is associated with (but not necessarily the cause of) mild depression, irritability, water retention, dysbiosis (and increased risk of candida), breast soreness, lowered libido and excessive sleepiness.

Testosterone helps with memory, mood and motivation (see page 165, for more information).

The key to your emotional and mental health is to get the balance of hormones right, but also to achieve the optimum ratio between them. It's now believed that oestrogen dominance is particularly prevalent among women and is a major contributor to a variety of hormone-related problems, such as PMS, endometriosis, fibroids and the menopause. In part, this is believed to be due to poor diet, stress and exposure to xeno-oestrogens (oestrogen-like chemicals found in pesticides, cling film, plastic bottles and fatty foods).

If you scored 12 or more on the oestrogen/progesterone imbalance questionnaire, you'd benefit from taking the following steps.

Get a saliva test

I would highly recommend getting a saliva test from a reputable laboratory to measure your hormone levels. You really need to know what levels and patterns of change in your hormone levels are present before selecting a treatment. (See Resources, page 282.)

Address the underlying causes of hormonal imbalance

The underlying causes of and contributors to oestrogen/progesterone imbalance might be:

- Poor diet (see below and Pillar Four)

- Stress (Pillar Six)

- Nutritional deficiencies (Pillars Four and Five)

- Hormone imbalances (Pillar Five)

- Excessive intake of alcohol and caffeine, smoking (addictions, Pillars Four and Six)

- Sleep deprivation (Pillar Four)

- Dysbiosis (Pillar Five)

- Lack of physical activity (Pillar Four)

- Toxicity (Pillar Five)

- Poor emotional management (Pillars One and Two)

- Not meeting your emotional needs (Pillar Three)

- Allergies (Pillar Five)

- Hypothyroidism (Pillar Five)

- Adrenal fatigue (Pillar Five)

- Electropollution (Pillar Four)

- Depression and anxiety (Pillar Six)

- Dysglycemia (Pillars Four and Five)

Hormone-based treatments

While the suggestions in this book usually do correct imbalances, you might need to take a hormone-based treatment; if so, I would encourage you to read my book *Holistic Health Secrets for Women*, which explores the issues of hormones in some depth. The key with hormone treatment is to take the minimum amount that will resolve your symptoms, and to do so for the shortest possible period of time, while regularly monitoring your hormone levels.

Note: hormone-based treatments should only ever be used under the guidance of a medical doctor.

Make dietary changes

- If your oestrogen levels are too low, the following foods can raise them naturally: apples, plums, cherries, coconut, tomatoes, potatoes, olives, yams, carrots and brown rice.

- If your oestrogen levels are too high, fermented soya foods, such as tempeh and miso can help to normalise them, as they contain genisteins (a type of phyto-oestrogen). Other phyto-oestrogens include apples, flaxseed, nuts, celery, wholegrains and alfalfa.

Take dietary supplements

- In addition to taking a multivitamin–mineral–antioxidant, vitamin C with bioflavonoids and fish oil/flaxseed oil (see Pillar

Four), you should also consider taking *Vitex agnus-castus* – this is one of the most widely recommended herbs for women who have symptoms relating to progesterone deficiency.[84] The usual dose is 4mg a day of a standardised extract.

- Black cohosh is commonly used to treat the symptoms of the menopause, such as hot flushes, sleep disturbances and sweating. It is also known to raise levels of the neurotransmitter serotonin, so is helpful if symptoms are accompanied by a depressed mood. How black cohosh works is unclear.[85] The usual dose is 20–40mg a day.

  Note: black cohosh should not be used if you have any pre-existing liver problems.

- Fermented soya products (use dose as advised by manufacturers) containing the equivalent amount of active isoflavones found in the average Japanese diet – about 40mg – are good for alleviating hot flushes.[86] (I tend to use them alongside black cohosh; see Resources, page 284.)

- Milk thistle and dandelion are herbs that work well in combination, helping to support optimum liver function and reduce circulating levels of oestrogen.

- Saw palmetto[87] (320mg of a standardised extract) is useful for reducing testosterone levels and treating excess hair growth and acne in polycystic ovary syndrome (PCOS) sufferers.

Testosterone imbalance (men)

This section is focused on testosterone levels as they relate to men. (Whereas testosterone levels do have a significant role to play in the health of women, I do not advocate treating testosterone imbalances without professional supervision.)

Testosterone is produced by the adrenal glands, and the testicles in men. It can have a significant effect on the way that you feel and on the health and growth of the body. It influences sex drive, calcium deposition in the bones, muscle growth, strength, stamina, red cell production and even cholesterol levels.[88] From the age of thirty onwards, levels of biologically active (free) testosterone start dropping at a rate of between 1 and 2 per cent a year, until the age of seventy. By the time a man reaches eighty, he has a one in two chance of having a testosterone level low enough to be causing health problems.

In men, low testosterone levels lead to reduced libido, motivation and energy, depression, deteriorating memory, excess weight around the middle, impotence, infertility, high cholesterol, soft erections and loss of muscle mass. With the obvious exception of the soft erections, the effects on women are similar.

My own experience with helping men with testosterone imbalances is that as long as the levels are being monitored, the advice below can be used safely and effectively. So, if you scored twelve or more on the men's testosterone questionnaire, you should take the following steps.

Get a saliva test

I would highly recommend getting a saliva test from a reputable laboratory to measure your hormone levels. You really need to know what levels and patterns of change in your hormone levels are present before selecting a treatment. (See Resources, page 282, for details of supplier.) If your test results show that you have low levels of testosterone, I would strongly encourage you to seek help from a medical doctor who has experience in male hormonal imbalances.

Address the underlying causes of testosterone imbalance

The underlying causes of, and contributors to, your testosterone imbalance might be:

- Poor diet (see below and Pillar Four)

- Stress (Pillar Six)

- Nutritional deficiencies (Pillars Four and Five)

- Hormone imbalances (Pillar Five)

- Excessive intake of alcohol and caffeine, smoking (addictions, Pillars Four and Six)

- Sleep deprivation (Pillar Four)

- Dysbiosis (Pillar Five)

- Lack of physical activity (Pillar Four)

- Toxicity (Pillar Five)

- Poor emotional management (Pillars One and Two)

- Not meeting your emotional needs (Pillar Three)

- Allergies (Pillar Five)

- Hypothyroidism (Pillar Five)

- Depression and anxiety (Pillar Six)

- Dysglycemia (Pillars Four and Five)

Testosterone replacement therapy

This is available on prescription or privately, and comes as patches, gel, capsules, oral lozenges, injections and implants. It's crucially important that you don't use any synthetic testosterone product (including methyltestosterone) as these have been associated with increased risk of cancer and liver problems.

Note: this treatment should only ever be taken under the care and direction of a medical doctor.

Take dietary supplements

- Zinc – 50mg helps to stop the conversion of testosterone into oestrogen, as well as helping to raise testosterone levels and boost sperm count. I usually recommend my patients take this for three months and then reduce it to 15mg a day. In one study, thirty-seven infertile men with decreased testosterone levels and associated low sperm counts were given 60mg of zinc daily for fifty days. In twenty-two of them, testosterone levels significantly increased and mean sperm count rose from 8 million to 20 million.[89]

- If you are taking testosterone replacement therapy you should also consider taking the herb saw palmetto, as this might help to reduce the risk of developing prostate problems. It works by inhibiting the enzyme that converts the testosterone into dehydrotestosterone, a hormone that stimulates prostate cell growth. It also blocks oestrogens and should be used alongside testosterone replacement therapy.[90]

Note: saw palmetto can interfere with PSA levels, a marker for prostate cancer and inflammation.

Dysbiosis

Our guts are teeming with over 100 trillion microscopic bacteria. When our immune system is strong and gut function intact, we live in harmony with these bacteria. We provide food, water and shelter and they, in turn, repay us by helping to develop and mature the immune system, manufacture vitamins, keep disease-promoting bacteria in check, aid recovery from infection, repair and promote the health of the digestive tract and reduce the severity of inflammatory conditions. When things are balanced and calm, all is well.

However, if our immune system weakens, because of stress or toxicity, or our gut function deteriorates because of mineral, stomach acid and/or digestive-enzyme deficiencies or we expose ourselves to steroids, NSAIDS or antibiotics, the situation reverses. Disease-promoting bacteria (such as certain strains of E. coli and Klebsiella) and other microbes, such as candida and parasites take hold and start to produce toxins, which interfere with the normal functioning of the digestive tract. This state of imbalance in which the normal healthy population of beneficial bacteria in the intestines has been disrupted is called dysbiosis and is believed to be an underlying factor in many health problems, such as foggy thinking, depression, obsessive compulsive disorder, mood swings, anxiety, low energy as well as rheumatoid arthritis, irritable bowel syndrome, ankylosing spondylitis and inflammatory bowel disease.[91]

Treating dysbiosis

The three main types of dysbiosis are fungal (including candida, the most common one in my patients), bacterial and parasitic. The three can co-exist.

If you scored 12 or more on the dysbiosis questionnaire, you'd benefit from taking the following steps.

Consult a nutritional therapist

To determine which type of dysbiosis you have, I highly recommend consulting with a nutritional therapist or integrative medical doctor (see Resources, pages 275–76), who can arrange a test called the comprehensive digestive stool analysis with parasitology (CDSAP) 2.0 test. Your practitioner will use the information from the test to decide which type you have; usually it's a combination. As a rule, you will need to treat it for a minimum of six months, maybe up to twelve.

While your practitioner will tailor a programme to your needs, here is an overview of how I go about treating the patients who come to see me.

Address the underlying causes of dysbiosis

The underlying causes of and contributors to your dysbiosis might be:

- Low probiotic levels (take a probiotic for six months)
- Low stomach acid and/or digestive enzyme levels (take a replacement supplement for one to two months)
- Poor diet (see below and Pillar Four)
- Nutritional imbalances (Pillars Four and Five)
- Stress (Pillar Six)
- Non-steroidal anti-inflammatories or steroids
- Excessive intake of alcohol and caffeine, smoking (addictions, Pillar Six)
- Inflammatory bowel disease
- Gut infection
- Constipation

Note: if you take antibiotics (which will kill the probiotics that you do have), make sure you take a course of probiotics afterwards.

Make dietary adjustments

- If you have a fungal dysbiosis, such as candida, you should for a minimum of six weeks avoid all sugar, as sugar feeds candida. This includes all sweets, chocolate, confectionary, soft drinks, cakes, puddings, desserts, jams, fruit juices, honey, molasses, fructose, maple syrup, corn syrup, sucrose, dried fruits and sweet fruits such as grapes, bananas, peaches and melon. You should also avoid white rice, white bread, white pasta and white flour products. Some people who are sensitive to candida can experience a cross-reaction with other yeasts. As a precaution I recommend avoiding the following yeast-containing foods and drinks: alcoholic drinks, pizza bases, vinegar, yeast extracts such as marmite, soy sauce, leavened bread, and stock cubes. You should also avoid moulds such as those found in Brie, blue cheese and Camembert. During this time you can eat plenty of vegetables, wholegrains, potatoes, eggs, meat, fish, dairy products (without sugar) and one portion of berries (such as blueberries, raspberries and blackberries), grapefruit, avocados or green apples a day, and then increase it to two portions after six weeks. The natural sweeteners xylitol, stevia and fructo-oligosaccharide (FOS), when used in moderation, are a healthy alternative to sugar. After six weeks, you can cautiously re-introduce sugar – although I suggest adopting a low-sugar diet for health reasons.

- In addition to taking a multivitamin–mineral–antioxidant, vitamin C with bioflavonoids and fish oil (3000–10,000mg) or flaxseed oil and an acidophilus and bifidobacterium-containing probiotic (Pillar Four), you should also consider taking the supplements and medications advised by your CDSAP 2.0 test; it will tell you which will work for you. Acidophilus and bifidobacterium types of probiotics are recognised as being two of the most important for health and well-being.

Fungal dysbiosis treatment plan

I tend to recommend either an anti-fungal medication, such as Diflucan (fluconazole) or nystatin and/or a combination of oregano, caprylic acid, thyme and pau d'arco and an oxygenated magnesium product. I use the latter with at least 80 per cent of my patients. I also tend to alkalise the body with alkaline mineral salts and support liver function with the herb milk thistle (see Resources, page 285, for more information).

To support your immune system, try taking a mix of organic mushroom tinctures or Biobran MGN-3 (a natural compound made from breaking down rice bran with enzymes from the shiitake mushroom; see Resources, page 278, for more information). Both of these activate the body's natural killer cells.

Bacterial dysbiosis treatment plan

The successful treatment of bacterial dysbiosis, the most common type of which is small intestinal bacterial overgrowth (SIBO), relies on eating a specialised diet, similar to that for fungal dysbiosis, while also taking a probiotic supplement and an antibacterial preparation. This can be either medication or a herbal product. The most common drug of choice for treating SIBO is neomycin and metronidazole. Herbal treatment options include grapefruit seed extract, garlic, ginger, olive leaf extract, berberine and echinacea. The exact ones you need to use will be determined by your CDSAP 2.0 results.

Parasitic dysbiosis treatment plan

This should only be done under supervision of an integrative medical doctor or nutritional therapist. In practice, most people with parasite infections need to be treated with anti-parasite medications. The results of the CDSAP 2.0 test will guide your doctor in choosing which medication to use. However, the most common and effective ones include metronidazole, paromomycin and doxycycline.

PILLAR FIVE: Summary

- Issues to do with emotional and mental health are not always psychological in origin.

- If you have a mood problem, consider whether it is influenced by any of the following: neurotransmitter, nutritional, blood-sugar, allergies, food intolerances, hormone imbalances, dysbiosis (gut flora imbalance), toxicity, medications, illness and structural problems.

- Exploring the possibility that you may have physical imbalances, and then taking action to address them, has the potential to make a real difference to your health and mood.

Pillar Six: Identify and address any mental-health challenges

Mental-health problems are on the increase. In 2001, the World Health Organization reported that worldwide there are 450 million people afflicted with a mental or neurological disorder.[92] What's more, few people will ever look for help, and of those who do, in my opinion, only a very small number will receive help that is tailored to them. Western medicine's approach to mental health and illness is short-sighted. While doctors and psychologists tend to be quite good at getting the diagnosis right, they often fail to search for the underlying causes, and diagnostic labels alone rarely tell us what these are.

My approach is different. When patients come to me with depression and/or anxiety, rather than prescribing medications and/or referring them for cognitive behavioural therapy (CBT), which is the standard medical approach, I work with them to identify the underlying barriers to them recovering, and this, I have found, is the key to lasting successful treatment (and emotional healing). Here are two case studies which demonstrate the importance of a personalised approach that deals with the root issues.

CASE STUDY: SONIA

Sonia was an executive who had been experiencing low-grade chronic depression for about three years. She had tried cognitive behavioural therapy with some initial success, but relapsed within two months. I noted that Sonia looked great and projected a strong, confident demeanour that belied her feelings of worthlessness and depression. After speaking with her for some time and having completed her questionnaires, I diagnosed one of the most important health problems that masquerade as depression – addictions. And if an individual is compulsively using alcohol, drugs, sex, shopping, work and so on, it is difficult to facilitate a lasting recovery from depression.

Sonia's treatment programme was divided into stages. Stage one involved complete abstinence from alcohol, regular attendance at Alcoholics Anonymous, a nutritional programme designed to nourish her body–mind and support her recovery (along the lines of Pillar Three), and training in mindfulness, meditation and stress management. This lasted for about twelve months, during which her depression lifted completely, while her physical health improved considerably. The second stage of treatment involved exploring issues of co-dependency (see page 245), as well as grief work and learning the skills of living, loving and relating. Although this work was challenging, Sonia thrived on it and, to this day, is leading a deeply fulfilling life because of the 'gift' of her depression.

CASE STUDY: THOMAS

When I first saw Thomas he was two stone overweight, had recently become unemployed and had been plagued by moderate severity depression for seven months. After a number of investigations, I was confident that biological and psychological factors were contributing to his experience. I started Thomas on a nutritional programme which included 5-HTP, high dose omega-3s, chromium and a B-complex. (There is some evidence that depression associated with weight gain, heavy arms/legs, cravings for sweets/carbohydrates and a feeling of grogginess responds very well to chromium.) He also reduced his intake of sugar considerably, stopped all caffeine and started a healthy-eating programme. He started an exercise programme through his local gym and, being an avid user of the Internet, he signed up with the free CBT course available on www.moodgym.anu.edu.au. (I have found this course to be very useful for patients who either don't want to or can't get to see a CBT therapist). However, the real key to Thomas's recovery, according to him, was the human potential coaching he received. By working with a human potential coach he was able to discover his strengths, values and talents, and from that place of self-awareness and insight start building a new career for himself. Within four weeks he had set up his own business, which has subsequently become very successful.

Thomas's depression lifted quickly, within two weeks. Furthermore – and this is one of the barometers by which I measure success – he started to develop a gratitude for life that he had never had before. In addition, he felt increasingly alive and confident that he had the resources to deal with 'whatever life brings his way'.

So there we have it: two people labelled with the same diagnosis, but with two very different pathways to recovery. There is a multitude of approaches that can work – I have had patients who have recovered from depression using acupuncture, hands-on healing, Human Givens therapy and spiritual healing – but the key, from my perspective as an integrative medical doctor, is to match the person and their health situation to the treatment (in the correct order) that is right for them.

In this pillar, I am going to outline my drug-free approach to the most common mental and emotional challenges that I see and diagnose in my patients:

- Psychological stress

- Anger

- Depression

- Anxiety and panic disorders

- Addictions

- Trauma/post-traumatic stress disorder (PTSD)

- Grief

To help you work out whether any of the above is relevant to you (most people have at least one), I provide here the same questionnaires that I use with my patients.

Mental-health questionnaires

These questionnaires aren't diagnostic of a problem, but a score of 12 or more is a strong indication that you'd benefit from addressing the area(s) in question along the lines suggested. Each question refers to the period of the last month. Take your time to read through and then fill in each of the questionnaires. Once you have done this, insert your totals into the score chart on page 182, or in your notebook or journal. Score the statements in each of the questionnaires in the following way:

No = 0, Occasionally = 1, Yes = 2

If you answer 'Yes' to a question where you see another score in brackets, use that score instead.

MENTAL HEALTH QUESTIONNAIRES

Psychological stress

Do you:

- Think stress is negatively influencing your health or quality of life? (score 6)

- Find it hard to cope with stressful situations?

- Have a low perseverance level?

- Experience irritability, worry and/or short temperedness? (score 6)

- Struggle to manage your stress?

- Believe that you don't have much control over your quality-of-life experience?

- Struggle to learn from or admit your mistakes?

- Manage stress through the use of food, drink, smoking, gambling, drugs or sex?

- Experience headaches, pounding heart, shortness of breath, muscle aches, unexplained back pain, clenched jaws, teeth grinding, stomach upsets, increased sweating, tiredness, sleep problems, weight gain/loss, sex problems, skin breakouts? ☐

- Experience anxiety, restlessness, worrying, irritability, depression, sadness, anger? ☐

- Experience mood swings, job dissatisfaction, burnout, forgetfulness, inability to concentrate? (score 6) ☐

Total score ☐

Anger

Do you:

- Experience explosive outbursts of anger and/or violence? ☐

- Tend to be impatient? ☐

- Have critical or resentful thoughts towards other people? ☐

- Experience tension in certain situations and/or hold tension in your body? ☐

- Get defensive around certain people, issues or situations? ☐

- Try to control people and/or try to persuade them to agree with you? ☐

- Have others telling you that you are blunt, insensitive and/or rude? ☐

- Tend to blame others? ☐

- Deliberately avoid sensitive or stressful subjects? ☐

- Tend to suffer from unexplained physical complaints, such as headaches and/or back pain? ☐

Total score ☐

Depression

Do you:

- Have a veil of sadness around you? (score 6) ☐

- Feel down, depressed or hopeless? ☐

- Have little interest or pleasure in doing things? ☐

- Experience fatigue or low energy? ☐

- Have problems with your sleep? ☐

- Experience feelings of agitation or a sense of intense slowness? ☐

- Experience a sense of guilt or worthlessness nearly all the time? ☐

- Know you are depressed? (score 12) ☐

- Have recurring thoughts of death or suicide? (score 6) ☐

- Take antidepressants? (score 12) ☐

Total score ☐

Anxiety and panic disorders

Do you:

- Worry continually almost every day about both big and small problems, situations, events and/or activities? ☐

- Have difficulty controlling your worries or anxieties? ☐

- Have trouble keeping your mind on one thing? ☐

- Feel restless or on edge much of the time? ☐

- Get easily irritable or angry? ☐

- Sometimes sweat or have a lump in your throat when you're worried? ☐

- Know you are anxious? (score 12) ☐

- Experience worrying that interferes with your normal routines, work or school and/or social activities? ☐

- Have an intense fear that you will do or say something that will embarrass you in front of other people? ☐

- Have a specific phobia? (score 6) ☐

  Total score ☐

Addictions

Do you:

- Suspect that you have an addiction? (score 12) ☐

- Have a persistent desire or a history of unsuccessful attempts to cut down or to control a particular substance, substances or activity? (score 12) ☐

- Find that your tolerance for a particular substance, substances or activity (food, drink, drug, sex, gambling, taking care of others, obsessing, smoking) is increasing? ☐

- Become unsettled at the thought of not being able to have the substance(s) or activity, if told that you couldn't have it or them? ☐

- Find yourself giving up or reducing important social, occupational or recreational activities because of the substance(s) or activity? ☐

- Continue with the substance(s) or activity despite the knowledge that a persistent or recurrent physical or psychological problem is likely to be caused or exacerbated by it? ☐

- Experience withdrawal symptoms from the substance(s) or activity? ☐

- Become jittery or anxious without a coffee, alcohol, cigarette or something sweet? ☐

- Smoke cigarettes? ☐

- Find that having had one alcoholic drink you have to have another one? (score 6) ☐

Total score ☐

Trauma/PTSD

Do you:

- Have a history of experiencing, witnessing or being exposed to one or more traumatic events? (score 6) ☐

- Think trauma is in any way limiting your quality of life and/or health? (score 6) ☐

- Recollect feeling intense fear, helplessness and/or horror during the traumatic event? ☐

- Regularly experience recurring or intrusive thoughts about a past traumatic event? ☐

- Have a history of being repeatedly exposed to physical, sexual, emotional, intellectual and or spiritual abuse? ☐

- Have a history of experiencing bullying, stalking or harassment? ☐

- Deliberately avoid certain situations, people, activities or conversations in order to avoid unpleasant feelings? ☐

- Have a history of invasive medical or dental procedures, severe illness, prolonged immobilisation or automobile accidents? ☐

- Recollect as a child, being left alone, neglected, abused, abandoned, traumatised or shocked, or exposed to a loud noise or frightening situation? (score 6) ☐

- Have anxiety, OCD, chronic fatigue syndrome, insomnia or unexplained pain? ☐

Total score ☐

Grief

Do you:

- Need help and advice on how to grieve? (score 12) ☐

- Find it hard to talk about or think about a deceased person without crying and/or the voice cracking up, even though it is at least a year since they died? (score 6) ☐

- Have the feeling that the death occurred yesterday, even though the loss took place months or years ago? ☐

- Find that you are unwilling to move the material possessions of the deceased? ☐

- Struggle to mourn the loss of someone close to you? ☐

- Feel significant emotional pain when you think of the deceased person? (score 6) ☐

- Feel that your childhood was in any way less than nourishing? ☐

- Wish that your life had been different in any way? ☐

- Think that you are in any way distracting yourself from processing grief, for example by overeating or using drugs and/or alcohol? (score 6) ☐

- Have a sense of shame or guilt around a particular loss? ☐

Total score ☐

Your scores

Having completed the questionnaires, the next step is to transfer your scores to the chart below or, if you prefer, to a notebook or journal. If you have scored over 12 in more than one, I'd recommend starting by addressing the one you scored highest on. If you select more than three, or are feeling overwhelmed, that is a sign that you should work with an experienced integrative medical doctor or other mental-health professional.

Imbalance	Your score
Psychological stress	☐
Anger	☐
Depression	☐
Anxiety and panic disorders	☐
Addictions	☐
Trauma/PTSD	☐
Grief	☐

Psychological stress

Stress is part and parcel of life. Without it, life would be boring and uninteresting; and indeed there is good evidence to suggest that we need a degree of stress to grow and evolve. But why does stress get such bad press and what exactly do we mean by psychological stress? Here are two of the most popular definitions of stress:

- Stress is the adverse reaction people have to excessive pressure or other types of demand placed on them.

- Stress occurs when pressure exceeds your perceived ability to cope.[93]

At the heart of these definitions lies the idea that what really determines whether something is positively or negatively stressful is your perception of it – your perspective and interpretation of the situation in which you find yourself.

Stress = unmet needs

In my own work, I have found it useful to think of the term stress as referring to the tension and emotional *dis*-ease that can be felt in the body when a need isn't being met. Stress is therefore an invitation to stop, feel what you are feeling, then take action to identify your unmet need. Remember, your emotions are related to what is going on in your mind, as well as your body, so it's important to think laterally about causes. For example, you might be experiencing tension because your blood sugar has dropped too low, or because you are sleep deprived or because you need some rest. At another time, you may experience stress because you are resisting reality, you haven't spoken your truth; or maybe you have a tendency to perfectionism and have set yourself an impossible deadline.

Here is a list of some of the main physical and psychological contributors to psychological stress:

Psychological contributors

Identification with negative thoughts

Fighting/resisting reality

Resisting impulse to grow and spiritually evolve

Seeking fulfilment in the outside world

Not respectfully speaking your truth

Not meeting your emotional needs

Self-limiting beliefs

Addictions, anxiety and/or trauma

Co-/counter-dependency

Emotional suppression/repression

Suppressing creativity

Low self-acceptance

Tendency to self-criticism and/or comparing

Tendency to perfectionism and/or control

Not being present, in the here and now

Black-and-white, all-or-nothing thinking

Feeling isolated or unsupported

Low emotional resilience (ability to adapt to a situation)

Lack of certain emotional-management skills

Lack of nature connection

Physical contributors

Adrenal fatigue

Poor diet

Excessive sugar consumption

Sleep deprivation

Excess alcohol, caffeine

Genetic inheritance/ vulnerability

Lack of rest/relaxation

Too little/too much exercise

Spine misalignment

Medication

Neurotransmitter imbalances

Nutritional imbalances

Dysglycemia

Hormone imbalance

Inflammation

Allergies and food intolerances

Toxicity

Lack of sunshine

Signs and symptoms of stress

The prerequisite for stress management is stress awareness – being able to recognise the signs and symptoms of stress. When you are used to being stressed and tense it can be quite hard to be aware of these; for this reason it's worth asking a close friend or partner what they notice when they see you are stressed. Some of the most common signs and symptoms are muscle tension, restlessness, mental distraction and feeling emotionally tense and uneasy.

Effects of stress on your body

Signals from your body that you are stressed include headache, pounding heart, shortness of breath, muscle aches, back pain, clenched jaws, tooth grinding, stomach upsets, increased sweating, tiredness, sleep problems, weight gain or loss, sex problems and skin breakouts.

Effects of stress on your thoughts and feelings

Stress can affect your thoughts and feelings through anxiety, restlessness, worrying, irritability, depression, sadness, anger, mood swings, job dissatisfaction, burnout, forgetfulness, inability to concentrate and seeing only the negatives.

Effects of stress on your behaviour

Stress most commonly manifests in behaviour through over/undereating, angry outbursts, drug abuse, excessive drinking, increased smoking, social withdrawal, relationship conflicts, decreased productivity and blaming others.

Effects of stress on your health

Chronic stress is a known contributor to depression, heart disease, poor immune health, increased deposition of fat around the abdomen, infertility, poor concentration and memory and raised cholesterol and triglycerides.

If you've noticed any of the above signs or symptoms, this may indicate that you would benefit from taking action to manage your stress.

If you scored 12 or more on the psychological stress questionnaire, you'd benefit from taking the following steps.

Read Pillars One and Two

I recommend that you start by reading through Pillars One and Two, as this will familiarise you with some important ideas about stress and emotion and provide you with some good tools.

Use 4/7 breathing

A useful and effective approach to try once you become aware of stress is to turn your attention immediately to your heart area and start using 4/7 breathing, in which you breathe in to the count of four and out to the count of seven (see page xxiii). Do this for a couple of minutes, then feel your emotion fully (see Cradling and EmoTrance, in Pillar Two, pages 53 and 55) and ask yourself, 'What do I need in order to bring my body–mind into balance?'

In my experience, this generally relates to the need to:

- Welcome the reality of the situation

- Speak your truth

- Express/process your emotion

- Eat, sleep or rest

- Make a decision or take positive practical action

Address underlying issues

If you experience ongoing or recurring patterns of stress, such as anxiety, depression, or anger, stress-reduction approaches will be limited in their effectiveness. What needs to happen is that the underlying issues, such as trauma, addictions, co- and counter-dependency and low self-acceptance are dealt with. The questionnaires in Part Two will help you identify those that are relevant.

Use reprogramming

If, for example, you emotionally overreact with anger to a fairly harmless comment by your partner, I would recommend that as well as dealing with the underlying causes of anger (see page 188), you try reprogramming your responses. This can be done in a number of ways including:

- Hypnotherapy

- Self-hypnosis

- Two approaches called Heart Lock-In and Freeze Frame, from the HeartMath Institute. (See Resources, page 285, for more information.)

Use stress-reduction tools

Use a stress-reduction tool each day, and as and when necessary. Here are some suggestions: core stress release (see below), listening to relaxing music (see Resources, page 285, where I've made a number of recommendations), qi gong (I highly recommend Spring Forest qi gong – see Resources, page 285), yoga, t'ai chi, meditation, five rhythms/movement medicine, prayer, walking in nature, taking a hot bath, using aromatherapy oils or Bach flower remedies (especially rescue remedy; see Resources, page 285) and massage.

EXERCISE: Core stress release

Stress and emotional tension are held within the body. Core stress release is an easy-to-learn series of exercises which increase emotional body awareness and body acceptance, while simultaneously releasing the deep muscle contractions and tension held in the emotional and physical body in response to stress and trauma. This is one of the most important tools that I use with patients who have anxiety, depression, emotionally induced pain and/or PTSD. Used daily, it's also a great way of discharging the build-up of stress and tension in the body.

To get the most benefit from it and get used to it I recommend that you use it for ten minutes each day for one to two weeks, then as needed thereafter; many people continue to use it daily.

- Make sure you will not be disturbed for the next ten minutes.

- Stand against the wall, so that your back is supported.

- Bend your knees and move both feet out in front of you, making sure your back is still supported by the wall and that you are still fairly comfortable. If this puts too much strain on your knees, move your feet closer to the wall and move your bottom up the wall; this will relieve the pressure.

- Next, while keeping your eyes open and looking slightly upwards, set an intention. Say silently, 'I allow my body to release any tension and trapped energy.'

- Now gently start bouncing up and down on your legs.

- After twenty seconds or so, stop making the bouncing/shaking happen and allow your body to continue with it (which it will do).

- The key is to allow the shaking to occur, while you just focus on your breathing – take deep breaths in and out. Become like a rag doll, allowing yourself to go floppy.

- Now allow the shaking to move up from your legs/thighs, into your pelvis, and on up into the rest of your body.

- Shake your arms and hands gently, then allow the body's natural shaking to take over.

- If you feel panicked or are worried about being 'out of control', just return your attention to taking deep breaths and this should settle.

- When your legs start to get tired, stand up straighter. Some people at this stage will stand away from the wall and allow the shaking to continue.

- After five or ten minutes, gradually and consciously reduce the shaking.

- Now stretch your muscles.

You might feel very energised afterwards or, as is more frequently the case, particularly for the first few sessions, you might feel tired. If the latter, take some time to rest. Occasionally, it can bring up strong emotions, during and afterwards. If they occur while doing the exercise, just continue and allow your body to release them; if they come up afterwards I recommend using EmoTrance (see page 53). If traumatic memories come up (this happens rarely) I would encourage you to seek the help of someone who is experienced with working with trauma (see page 204 and Resources, page 287, for more information).

Anger

If you scored 12 or more on the anger questionnaire this section is for you.

When was the last time you got angry? How did it make you feel inside? Were you scared of the energy of your anger or overwhelmed by it? Were you in control of it, or was it in control of you? Would it have been obvious to others that you were angry, or do you tend to hide away your anger? Maybe you reveal it in other ways by being critical, aloof, resentful, impatient, tense or sarcastic?

Getting clarity about the way you relate to anger and learning how to harness its energy is a liberating experience and an important part of moving towards true happiness. However, managing anger in a healthy way is a challenge for most people.

What is anger?

Anger is a completely normal, healthy emotion that is intimately connected to self-preservation – your need to protect yourself physically, emotionally, intellectually and spiritually. When someone invades or abuses these boundaries, anger firstly lets you know that this has happened and secondly it provides you with the energy, focus and motivation to do something about it. So, although anger is commonly thought of as being a negative emotion, it's not; what determines whether anger is healthy or not is the way that you deal with it.

If you use the energy of anger to empower you to make decisions, assert yourself in a respectful way, protect your boundaries and take positive constructive action, then that's a healthy use and expression of your emotion. However, if anger is suppressed or used to control, manipulate or hurt others and/or yourself, it's being expressed in a way that is unhealthy.

What is your anger style?

In addition to anger repression and suppression there are two main ways of expressing anger. As you read through the characteristics of each, see which most accurately describes how you relate to anger.

Openly aggressive anger

This is what most people think of as anger; it's the overt display of anger. Openly aggressive behaviours might include: making threats, physical and/or intellectual bullying, shouting, physical/sexual abuse, making derogatory remarks, hitting, raging, criticising, being sarcastic, bickering, answering back, needing to be right, being excessively self-centred and selfish, destroying things (objects, hurting animals etc.) and manic behaviour (walking, speaking, working or driving too fast).

Passive–aggressive anger

A person who uses a passive–aggressive style is aware of feeling angry, but because of fear they resort to covert, rather than overt ways of showing it. They often find it very hard to admit to others and sometimes to themselves that they are angry. Passive–aggressive behaviours might include: turning up late, keeping quiet, letting people down, 'forgetting' to do something, sulking, lying, provoking the other in order to trigger their anger, playing the victim, communicating in mixed messages, procrastinating, doing things slowly or to a low standard, doing something half-heartedly, complaining about someone behind their back (but not talking to them directly) and agreeing to do things, but then not doing them.

How to manage your anger

One of the keys to managing anger is to learn how to deal with it in the moment; but even more important is to explore and address any underlying causes or contributors to your anger. Here are some suggestions to help you with that.

Check for trauma

If the intensity of anger that you are feeling is disproportionate to what the situation warrants – for example your partner makes a harmless comment and you fly off the handle – it suggests you have either been repressing/suppressing resentments and frustrations in relationship to them and/or you are transferring anger that belongs to someone else (your parents, for example) on to them. Either way, I'd strongly encourage you to read the sections on trauma/PTSD (see page 202).

Check for underlying physical imbalances

This is definitely not one to leave out, especially if your anger tends to be explosive. If you haven't already, I would encourage you to fill in the questionnaires in Pillar Five to identify whether any of the following are contributing to your anger: neurotransmitter imbalances, nutritional imbalances, allergies (especially food intolerances), hormonal imbalances and heavy metal toxicity.

Calm yourself

It takes quite a bit of practice and time to master catching the anger as it arises, but as you start to become aware of potential triggers and early warning signs you'll get much better at it. The following are some suggestions for keeping yourself relatively calm.

Breathe deeply   This is by far the most important and simplest approach. I recommend 4/7 breathing (see page xxiii). Simply turn your attention to your belly, then breathe in to the count of four and out to the count of seven. Continue until you feel calmer. See the psychological stress section (page 182) for more suggestions.

Count   Combine this with the deep breathing. Count slowly from ten down to one and, if you can, visualise yourself walking down a spiral staircase, with each number representing a step. As you go down, experience yourself getting more calm.

Visualise   Breathe deeply and see your anger/frustration as a red liquid draining out of your body, through your feet into the ground below.

Safely discharge your anger Try twisting a towel, screaming, punching a pillow, screaming into a pillow. The key, when doing any of these, is to allow the energy of anger to be discharged, but to do so as a mature adult. Do this by standing with an upright posture and not losing yourself in your anger; allow it to come out, while being aware of it doing so. You should not do any of these in front of anyone (the exception being a therapist).

Learn how to be assertive
Using the energy of anger in a way that allows you to communicate respectfully, clearly and maturely can have a very positive impact on your self-confidence and relationships. See page 260 in Pillar Eight for information on developing assertiveness.

Depression

The prevalence of depression is rising worldwide every year and it is predicted to be the world's second-most common cause of disabling disease (after heart disease) by 2020.

Are you depressed?

The brief screening questionnaire at the beginning of this pillar is designed to alert you to the possibility that you might be experiencing depression. If you score 12 or more, you should consult with your doctor in order to have the diagnosis confirmed and medical causes of depression excluded. These include post-viral illness, cancer (for example cancer of the pancreas can present as depression), sleep apnoea, thyroid disease, Addison's disease, Cushing's disease, hyperparathyroidism, systemic lupus erythematosus, multiple sclerosis, stroke, addictions, alcohol and alcohol withdrawal, stimulant withdrawal and side effects of certain medications, such as steroids, cimetidine, blood-pressure-lowering medication, anxiolytics and digoxin.

Your GP will probably then assess the severity of your depression. To find out how bad your depression is, your doctor first looks for one of the three key symptoms which are:

- Feeling sad or low most of the time

- Losing interest in things you used to enjoy

- Having no energy or feeling really tired

A depressed person will have at least one of these symptoms on most days, most of the time, for two weeks. If you have a key symptom, your doctor will consider how many, if any, of the following symptoms you also have:

- Problems sleeping, or sleeping too much

- Poor concentration or difficulty making decisions

- Low self-confidence

- Poor or increased appetite

- Thoughts of suicide

- Agitation or sluggishness

- Feelings of guilt for no reason

A doctor usually decides that someone with four of these symptoms has mild depression; someone with five or six has moderate depression and someone with all of them has severe depression.

What causes depression?

The answer to this will depend on who you talk to. A doctor will probably say it's related to a genetically inherited vulnerability and an imbalance in your brain neurotransmitters; a nutritional therapist might say it's because of nutrient deficiencies, hormonal imbalances and/or food intolerances; a counsellor may say it's due to addictions, low self-acceptance or trauma; and a cognitive behavioural therapist might say it's down to the negative, 'black-and-white' way a person interprets their life circumstances.

From my own experience of having worked with hundreds of people with depression, the answer is that it depends on the individual. The key is to work out which factors are relevant to you.

How to deal with depression

If you scored 12 or more on the depression questionnaire, you'd benefit from taking the following steps.

Visit your GP

Go to your GP to get the diagnosis confirmed, then explore the options available to you. For severe depression you might want to consider antidepressants, for mild to moderate depression you will probably be given lifestyle advice (such as exercise) and a referral to see a cognitive behavioural therapist or a recommendation for an online CBT programme (see Resources, page 285).

One important review of studies relating to antidepressants and their effectiveness found that they do help severely depressed people, but for people with mild to moderate depression their effect is entirely that of a placebo, i.e. they work through belief and expectation. For this reason, I encourage most of my patients with mild to moderate depression to try the suggestions below prior to taking antidepressants.

Address the underlying causes of depression

Once you have a diagnosis, my advice is to work with someone who will be able to help you to address any underlying causes, contributors and triggers listed below. (If you are creating your own programme, I suggest you start with Pillars Five and One. After that Pillars Two, Three and Four.)

- Sleep deprivation (Pillar Four)

- Lack of sunlight (Pillar Four)

- Neurotransmitter imbalances, especially serotonin and dopamine (Pillar Five)

- Addictions (Pillar Six; this is a commonly missed cause of depression)

- Trauma/PTSD (Pillar Six)

- Co-/counter-dependency (Pillar Eight)

- Emotional suppression/repression (Pillars One and Two)

- Unmet emotional needs (Pillar Three)

- Stress (Pillar Six)

- Medication (Pillar Five)

- Illness (Pillar Five)

- Hormone imbalances (especially adrenal fatigue and hypothyroidism, Pillar Five)

- Dysglycemia (Pillars Four and Five)

- Toxicity (Pillar Five)

- Allergies (especially food intolerances, Pillar Five).

Tools and techniques
My recommended tools and techniques for depression are core stress release (page 186) and EmoTrance (page 53). Breathwork (page 56) is also appropriate but it needs to learned from a practitioner.

Take dietary supplements
My recommended supplements for depression include the foundation supplement programme described in Pillar Four and/or the supplements recommended for any physical imbalances you have (see Pillar Five). In addition to this, if your depression is associated with weight gain, heavy arms/legs, cravings for sweets/carbohydrates and a feeling of grogginess, take 600mcg of chromium a day.

Work with a professional
If you want to work with someone who can teach you how to manage your thinking and emotions more effectively, you might want to choose a practitioner of Human Givens therapy, acceptance and commitment therapy, cognitive behavioural therapy or solution-focused brief therapy (see Resources, page 285).

Online courses

You could try an online depression-management course. There are many different programmes for recovering from depression, but the two that my patients like most and which I'd recommend can be found at www.clinical-depression.co.uk and www.moodgym.anu.edu.au.

The Alpha-Stim SCS

Not everyone wants to deal with the underlying issues of their depression; for such patients I usually recommend a medical device called the Alpha-Stim SCS. It's a portable device that sends minute and painless electrical currents into the body. It's been shown in a number of clinical trials to relieve significantly in the majority of users the symptoms of depression, and most of my patients have benefited considerably from using it (see Resources, page 285).

For seasonal affective disorder (SAD)

If you've been diagnosed with SAD, consider purchasing a light box. Regular exposure to full-spectrum lighting can result in a significant improvement within just a couple of weeks (see Resources, page 286).

Anxiety and panic disorders

Anxiety is a normal response to stress or danger; it increases your ability to focus, helps you prepare for action and can improve your performance. A certain amount of anxiety, on occasions and when appropriate is very much part of being human. However, anxiety becomes a problem when it is experienced intensely and/or when it interferes with your ability to carry out tasks and live life fully.

Many of my patients experience a low-grade anxiety, a constant background worrying or need to control, but few recognise it as anxiety, mainly because they have been living that way for many years. It's usually when the anxiety becomes unbearable, because of a significant stress or hormonal shift (such as entering the perimenopause) that they seek help.

Interestingly, some of the most so-called 'together', dynamic and high-achieving people I meet have chronic anxiety, usually dating back to childhood. Having an anxious parent or parents, experiencing abuse, trauma or neglect as a child, being brought up in an environment where you don't feel safe and having a temperament in which you are predisposed to worrying can all lead to the experience of anxiety.

Types of anxiety

There are a number of different types of anxiety, all of which can overlap.

Generalised anxiety disorder

This is characterised by anxiety symptoms that are present much of the time and not related to any particular situations. It's experienced as an undercurrent of anxiety and worry and is often experienced by people with depression and phobias. It affects about 10 per cent of people, two thirds of whom are women.[94]

Panic disorder

This is marked by severe and often unpredictable panic attacks. Symptoms are extreme and include the feeling of dying, excessive hyperventilation and the fear of losing control or going mad.

Phobias

A phobia is a fear that is out of proportion to the situation that causes it and cannot be explained away. The person typically avoids the feared situation, since this helps to reduce the anxiety. Symptoms can include extreme anxiety, palpitations, tremors and dizziness.

Post-traumatic stress disorder (PTSD)

This can start any time after a traumatic incident either when someone perceives themselves to be in danger, that their life is being threatened or where they see others dying or being injured. Women are vulnerable to PTSD following childhood abuse, sexual abuse, rape, and traumatic childbirth. Symptoms include flashbacks and nightmares, intrusive thoughts and memories, insomnia, anger, numbness, depression, avoidant behaviour and being hypervigilant.

Obsessive compulsive disorder (OCD)

Although 14 per cent of the population experience minor obsessive symptoms, about 0.1 per cent of the population actually have OCD. Symptoms include obsessive thoughts, which are often disturbing and unpleasant and which the sufferer can't stop, which in itself adds to the stress. The obsessive thoughts can lead to compulsive, repetitive actions, for example repeated cleaning of hands or checking that the door is locked. Although the actions are not normally pleasurable, they reduce the experience of inner tension and decrease the obsessive thinking.

Treating anxiety

In my experience, treating anxiety needs to go beyond just reducing the symptoms. Anxiety, like most health challenges, is an invitation to grow up and wake up.

If you scored 12 or more on the anxiety questionnaire, you'd benefit from taking the following steps.

Visit your GP

If you suspect that you might be experiencing anxiety, you should be formally assessed by your GP to confirm the diagnosis. It is important to have various medical conditions also excluded, particularly if you suddenly develop anxiety out of the blue and are younger than eighteen or older than thirty-five. These include: hyperthyroidism, hypoparathyroidism, hypoglycaemia, neurological illness, addictions, toxicity, as well as medication side effects or withdrawal from medications, alcoholism or alcohol withdrawal, stimulants (such as cocaine and amphetamines), nicotine withdrawal and caffeine intoxication or withdrawal.

Address underlying causes

Once you have a diagnosis, my advice is to work with someone who can help you address any other underlying causes of, and contributors to, your anxiety – these are listed below. (If you are creating your own programme, you should start with Pillars Five and One, then go on to Pillars Two, Three and Four.)

- Neurotransmitter imbalances, especially GABA (Pillar Five)

- Addictions (Pillar Six)

- Trauma/PTSD (Pillar Six)

- Poor emotional management (Pillars One and Two)

- Unmet emotional needs (Pillar Three)

- Stress (Pillar Six)

- Hormone imbalances (Pillar Five)

- Dysbiosis (especially candida, Pillar Five)

- Excessive intake of alcohol and caffeine (Pillar Four)

- Smoking (addictions, Pillar Six)

- Dysglycemia (Pillar Five)

- Sleep deprivation (Pillar Four)

- Medications (Pillar Five)

- Illness (Pillar Five)

- Toxicity (Pillar Five)

- Allergies (Pillar Five)

Take dietary supplements
I recommend the foundation supplement programme described in Pillar Four and/or those suggested for any physical imbalances (Pillar Five). In addition, if you have a phobia, you might want to consider using the rewind technique (see page 205 and Resources, page 286).

Tools and techniques
Recommended tools and techniques are Core Stress Release (page 186), Cradling (page 55) and EmoTrance (page 53). Breathwork (see page 56) is also useful.

Work with a professional

If you want to work with someone who can help you to manage your thinking and emotions more effectively, you might want to choose a practitioner of Human Givens therapy, acceptance and commitment therapy, cognitive behavioural therapy or solution-focused brief therapy. (See Resources, page 285.)

The Alpha-Stim SCS

Not everyone wants to deal with the underlying issues of their anxiety, so for these patients I usually recommend a medical device called the Alpha-Stim SCS. It's a portable device that sends minute and painless electrical currents into the body. In clinical trials it's been shown to relieve symptoms of anxiety in the majority of users, and most of my patients have benefited considerably from using it. (See Resources, page 285.)

Addictions

So what exactly is an addiction? I define it as the compulsive use of any substance, activity or behaviour that is beyond your control and affects your health and life (and usually other people's) for the worse. Any recurring pattern of behaviour that is rooted in denial, dishonesty and/or secrecy and removes you from reality, responsibilities or relationships may indicate an underlying addiction.

One way I help my own patients understand compulsive behaviours – whether they are related to alcohol, drugs, nicotine, prescribed medications, or to food, sex, relationships, smoking, gambling, overspending, shopping, work or busyness – is this. It's to regard them as unskilled strategies for sedating, avoiding and controlling the emotional distress and tension that they are experiencing because they are failing to actively process these emotions. It is true that genetic factors and neurotransmitter and nutritional imbalances (and the other mental-health issues) contribute to the distressing emotions that lead to addictive behaviour. However, although these factors do need to be addressed, the major task for anyone with addictions is to change the way they are living their life.

If you have an addiction, this means making changes in the way you act, what you focus on and, importantly, changing the way you relate to yourself, to others and to life. The key is to face reality, grow up and proactively start creating a healthy, happy, and fulfilling life that is rooted in balance and moderation. Addiction recovery is therefore about much more than just abstaining from the behaviour of choice.

Treating addictions

Admitting to yourself and others that you have an addiction, and that you need help, is a significant step forward in your recovery programme. What you do next depends on what addictive tendencies are present, the severity of the situation, your existing physical, emotional and psychological level of health, your financial resources, your life circumstances, the impact on your family and the immediate risk of your problems. For this reason, I recommend that you work with an experienced addictions doctor or counsellor (see Resources, page 287).

While there are many different approaches to addiction recovery and a whole host of theories as to what causes addiction, I have found that a personalised holistic approach provides the greatest depth of recovery, healing and personal transformation. Rather than just using a medical or psychological approach to addiction treatment, I use an eclectic mix of nutritional, psychological, medical, social and spiritual approaches that are personalised to you. (To find out more, visit my website; see Resources, page 287.)

If you scored 12 or more on the addictions questionnaire or you think you have some addictions, here are my suggestions to get you started.

Identify your addictive tendencies
I mentioned this way back in the introduction, but if you haven't already, I encourage you to identify your addictive tendencies by filling in the in-depth online questionnaire at www.s-p-q.com. In my experience most people with addictions have at least three or four addictive behaviours including addiction to work, exercise, nicotine,

alcohol, shopping, Internet/gaming, sex, food, drugs, gambling, prescription drugs, love, compulsive overspending and so on.

Consider a residential programme

If your addictions are spiralling out of control, and/or if you are at risk of withdrawal symptoms due to consumption of alcohol or drugs, you will need to be assessed for either an inpatient or outpatient treatment programme which may or may not include detoxification (see Resources, page 286). Most treatment programmes last between 30 and 90 days. Ninety days plus is the optimum for most people.

Healthy self-care and dietary supplements

The areas that get neglected most in addiction treatment and recovery are healthy self-care and the use of diet and nutritional supplementation to reduce cravings, support detoxification, correct physical imbalances, improve mood and transform health. Many of the suggestions and recommendations in Pillars Three and Four cover these areas. The most common food intolerances/sensitivities that I find in my addiction patients are those to wheat, dairy and sugar.

Twelve-step support groups

Twelve-step support groups, such as Alcoholics Anonymous, Narcotics Anonymous and so on, can be invaluable for many people with addictions. They are based on a set of guiding principles for recovery from addictive, compulsive, or other behavioural problems. Those principles include admitting that you cannot control your addiction or compulsion; recognising a greater power that can give you strength and guidance; examining past errors with the help of a sponsor (experienced member); making amends for these errors; learning to live a new life with a new code of behaviour; and helping others who suffer from the same addictions or compulsions. Many people who attend these groups find them to be an important source of support and inspiration.

CBT hypnotherapy

If you are looking to give up nicotine, I have found that this specialised approach to hypnotherapy can help. The NHS Smoke-Free website also has some useful information, as does my own blog which you can access via my website (see Resources, page 287).

SMART recovery

SMART or self-management and recovery training is a not-for-profit organisation offering free support groups and online meetings through which you can learn about how to increase self-acceptance, self-reliance, self-motivation and manage urges, thoughts, feelings and behaviour. Unlike most approaches to addictions, which view them as a disease, SMART sees them as habits, which can be changed. If you do use this, my recommendation is to do so in conjunction with the twelve-step model. (See Resources, page 286, for more information.)

Note: if you are the partner of someone who has an addiction, please see my recommended books and websites in the Resources section.

Trauma/post-traumatic stress disorder (PTSD)

I have yet to work with anyone whose level of emotional health, quality of life and relationships haven't in some way been negatively influenced by trauma. Trauma is very much part and parcel of life, and learning how to recognise and recover from it is an essential part of moving towards a higher level of happiness and emotional health.

What is trauma?

Trauma refers to the debilitating symptoms experienced when our body–mind is unable to respond fully and effectively to a situation that we find threatening and overwhelming. I divide trauma into two types: developmental trauma, which is inflicted on children by their caregivers (this is covered in the co- and counter-dependency section on page 245) and shock trauma, which relates to a specific trauma-inducing event or events. What determines whether a person experiences an event as being traumatic or not depends not so much on the characteristics of the traumatic event itself, but their response to it. This, in turn, is related to a whole host of factors including age (children are very susceptible), emotional resilience, mental health, coping abilities, temperament, availability of support and past trauma history. So, while approximately 51–69 per cent of the population will encounter a shock trauma event in their life, only one third will actually go on to experience symptoms severe enough to warrant a diagnosis of PTSD.

PTSD

This develops after exposure to one or more terrifying events in which grave harm occurred or was threatened, and in response to which intense fear, helplessness or horror were experienced. It causes flashbacks, nightmares, a state of hyperarousal (involving problems sleeping and relaxing) and has a significant impact on health and relationships. People with PTSD often feel chronically numb and emotionally disconnected.

What events can trigger trauma?

Most of us, quite understandably, tend to associate trauma with obvious events, such as experiencing or witnessing physical or sexual abuse, experiencing or witnessing violence, war, natural disasters, accidents, major illness or the loss of a loved one. Indeed, one study interviewed women from five different countries and found that over a lifetime, up to 66 per cent of women had experienced physical abuse, 37 per cent emotional abuse and 33 per cent sexual abuse.[95] Other studies have found that 25 per cent of children experienced one or more forms of physical violence during childhood, 18 per cent experienced humiliation and/or attacks on self-esteem and 16 per cent of children aged under sixteen experienced sexual abuse during childhood.[96] The latter figure might even be conservative, as there is evidence that up to one in three incidents of child sexual abuse is not remembered by adults who experienced it as children.[97]

However, trauma can also happen after childbirth, minor injuries, witnessing a road traffic accident, panic attacks (where the person thinks they are going to die), medical procedures, injuries and minor illness. I have also found that many of my patients have experienced trauma through moving house as a child, starting a new school, watching traumatic scenes on TV, living with an emotionally, physically, intellectually or spiritually abusive person or experiencing a relationship break-up.

The consequences of trauma

These are sometimes obvious, but often also quite subtle. Few people will make the connection between the emotional neglect (which is trauma) they experienced as a baby, with the low self-esteem, problems with intimacy and addictions they experience as an adult. What's more, it's not just trauma per se that contributes to health problems; many people with trauma self-medicate their emotional pain with a variety of unhealthy behaviours, such as excessive consumption of alcohol and smoking cigarettes. All of these are known to impact negatively on well-being and quality of life.

Here are just some of the many effects and consequences of trauma: addiction, anxiety, chronic fatigue syndrome, fibromyalgia, depression, migraines, IBS, insomnia, low self-esteem, loss of confidence, unexplained chronic pain, nightmares, OCD, phobias and relationship problems.[98]

Overall, trauma impacts most greatly on the quality of life that a person is experiencing, with health, relationships, work and confidence being the most badly affected.

Treating trauma

If you scored 12 or more on the trauma/PTSD questionnaire, the following is relevant to you. There are many different treatments for people with trauma, and knowing which is going to be best for you can be difficult.

Work with an experienced practitioner

In my experience the most comprehensive and effective approach to trauma recovery involves working with an experienced practitioner with whom you feel safe and, importantly (I believe), has a variety of different tools and approaches under their belt, so that they can tailor your treatment to you. These are the four most common approaches.

The rewind technique   Also known as the fast phobia cure, the rewind technique is the approach with which my patients have experienced greatest success in respect of alleviating symptoms relating to post-traumatic stress disorder. The rewind technique is a safe, non-voyeuristic and highly effective method for treating trauma and PTSD. The vast majority of people experience a significant (over 70 per cent) reduction in their symptoms following one session. The process is gentle, comfortable and doesn't involve the 'reliving' of unpleasant events. (See Resources, page 286.)

EMDR   Eye movement desensitisation and reprocessing, or EMDR, is one of the most effective and intensively researched trauma therapies. It uses a series of eye movements or auditory stimuli to activate repeatedly the opposite sides of the brain, releasing emotional experiences that are 'trapped' in the nervous system. As troubling images and feelings are processed by the brain via the eye-movement patterns of EMDR, resolution of the issues and a more peaceful state are achieved. It is believed that the eye movements induced in EMDR mirror the natural eye-movement process that occurs in the REM phase of sleep, during which information is processed naturally. (See Resources, page 287.)

Somatic experiencing   Developed by the pioneering psychologist Peter Levine, SE works directly with body wisdom in a way that gently allows for the discharge and completion of the instinctual survival energies, resulting in a restored sense of settling and well-being. (See Resources, page 287 for more details.)

Trauma-release process   This is a body-based technique that activates the body's own trauma-resolution process in order to release deeply held tension patterns. Developed by David Berceli, an expert in the area of trauma intervention and conflict resolution, it can also be used effectively to release anger, anxiety and fear. I highly recommend it. (See Resources, page 291.)

For minor traumas

For minor traumas such as arguments (although these can be quite traumatic), I tend to use EmoTrance (page 53). Other sections that are relevant to trauma are 'Investigate your thinking' (page 28), Anger and Grief (page 188 and below).

Grief

Grief isn't something we feel solely when we lose someone we love, though of course this is one of the most raw experiences of grief. Grief is a natural emotional response to the experience of loss so, for example, the end of a relationship, the onset of health problems, or changes (such as starting a new school, travel or moving home) can all trigger grief. Many of us also hold grief 'energy' in relationship to the early years of our life.

We can also have grief over the life we have lived and the life we haven't lived – the discrepancy between how life should have been and how it actually has been. The gap between reality and the 'dream' can cause considerable pain and suffering; that is until the energy is processed and grieved. Some of my patients, especially those in addiction recovery, go through a process of grieving when they start to get in touch with the pain and tension they have been carrying in their bodies.

The grieving process

Grieving is the process by which trapped energy relating to a loss or series of losses is processed to the extent that it no longer limits your capacity for a healthy and fulfilling life. It is very much about making peace with and gaining a sense of completion around the loss. However, the path you take and the experience that you have will really depend on you, as there is no correct way to grieve. That said, I urge you not to rely on time, for time alone does not heal. Only knowledge and actions support healing.

The psychiatrist Elizabeth Kubler-Ross has done a lot of work around the process of dying and the response to significant or catastrophic loss.[99] She created a framework to help people through the process of grieving using a five-stage model:

1. **Denial** This is often accompanied by emotional numbness and a disbelief as to what has actually happened.

2. **Anger** This can be directed towards yourself, others and/or God, and is often accompanied by a variety of fears.

3. **Bargaining** 'What if' or 'if only' scenarios; guilt might also arise.

4. **Depression** Feeling intensely sad and depressed.

5. **Acceptance** Acceptance of the reality of the loss.

Of course, there is no typical response to loss and not everyone will go through the five stages or go through them in order. The purpose of the model is simply to provide the individual going through a loss with the knowledge and tools to support the process.

Signs and symptoms of unresolved grief

Signs and symptoms that may indicate you have unresolved grief include:

- Lack of present-moment awareness and problems with concentration
- Emotional withdrawal and isolation
- Disrupted sleeping and eating patterns
- Tiredness and fatigue
- Saying you are fine or OK after a significant loss
- Emotional numbness or outbursts of anger
- Feeling you are on an emotional rollercoaster
- Being excessively busy
- Feeling that you need to cry, but not allowing yourself to do so
- Blaming others for your loss
- Feelings of resentment
- Allowing your life and life decisions to be directed by fear
- Addictive behaviours

Suggestions for processing grief

If you scored 12 or more on the grief questionnaire, the following is relevant to you. The key to grieving is to take action. Here are some suggestions to support you on your journey.

Read Pillars One and Two

Rather than thinking your way through the process of loss and grieving, try feeling your way through. The suggestions in Pillar Two will help you with this. I also recommend reading the sections on defusing your negative thoughts and investigating your thinking (see pages 25 and 28). Both of these will show you how to be at peace with any stress-inducing thoughts you might be experiencing.

Crying

Crying can be an effective way to release stuck energy in the body. In my experience, the deepest healing from crying occurs when you cry in the presence of someone with whom you feel safe and, as you cry, you gently talk about what you are feeling and thinking.

Breathwork

A powerful way to integrate grief is through the use of Breathwork (see Pillar Two, page 56). However, this has to be learned from an experienced practitioner.

Talk/feel your way through your fears

Fears, such as the fear of the unknown, of death or of change often come up in the grieving process. Talk through these fears with a friend/family member or use one of the emotional-processing tools, such as Cradling (page 55) or EmoTrance (page 53) to help you.

Communicate your feelings

Do this as best you can to those who want to help you. See Honest Self-expression (Pillar Two, page 56).

Attend a seminar

Try attending a grief recovery seminar where you will learn effective tools for getting through the process (see Resources, page 287).

Tools and techniques

- Write a letter or try role-play scenarios relating to your grief in which you feel able to say the things you wish you had said or want to say now. Communication of unexpressed emotion and thoughts is an important part of the healing process.

- Process your emotions and emotional pain using any of the emotional-processing skills, such as Cradling or EmoTrance (pages 55 and 53). You might need to work with a practitioner if you find these hard to use yourself.

Consult a professional

If the grief relates to your childhood, consider working with a therapist or going on a workshop (see co-dependency/counter-dependency work providers, Resources, page 288).

PILLAR SIX: Summary

- A significant proportion of the population has suffered, or will suffer from mental ill-health at some time.

- Most people struggle with stress and anger.

- Drug-free approaches to mental health should be considered either alongside medication or as an alternative (if supervised).

- Failure to identify and address addictions, trauma and grief is a common reason why a high level of happiness is not experienced.

Part Three

Maximise your happiness

Pillar Seven: Accept and love yourself

This book is all about helping you to discover true happiness. It is something that you – that everyone – can experience, regardless of how you feel now. That may sound like a bold claim, but it is true and the reason is this: true happiness exists within us, we just have to take the actions that will enable us to experience it. You have learned many ways to do this in the previous pillars. However, they will only take you so far without one vital piece of the jigsaw – the ability to love and accept yourself.

Ninety per cent of the people who come to me lack self-acceptance and self-love. This lack is felt as a 'hole in the soul', a sense of emptiness within themselves. It's the deep existential pain of having lost sight of the knowledge that you are loved and loveable – that at the deepest level you are your true self, that you are love itself. And like someone who is looking for their car keys in their garden, when the keys are sitting on a table in their hallway, many of us go looking for love in the wrong place. We turn to partners, our parents, our work or to control, alcohol, food, drugs, prescription medications, work, sex and numerous other 'fillers' to provide the love we seek, yet, as we all know in our own experience, none of them truly provides the fulfilment that we need. How can they, when our love resides within our own hearts?

The self-acceptance solution

Take a couple of slow deep breaths and say to yourself, 'I deeply and completely accept and love myself, just as I am.' How does your body respond? Do you feel peaceful, light and expanded, or tense, contracted and heavy? Do you genuinely accept and love yourself, or do you not?

To some people this sounds like a bizarre thing to do. It can sound self-indulgent, self-centred and unnecessary. One patient of mine protested that if he accepted and loved himself, he would no longer be a man. A man, as he went on to say, 'needs spine and vision, not a soft heart'. In truth, and as I told him, for true happiness and peace of mind we need both 'spine' (whereby we speak truthfully and act with integrity) and 'heart' (the capacity for acceptance, love and compassion, both for ourselves and others). We also need 'guts' – the ability to act courageously and to do so despite our fears. It's a question of balance.

So, how can we open our hearts and experience true intimacy and love? One way, and the way I am going to explain here, is through self-acceptance and self-love.

What are self-acceptance and self-love?

Self-acceptance is the process of bringing an inner acceptance to the reality, right now of every part of you, warts and all. When you unconditionally accept yourself, you see all the different aspects of yourself – thoughts, feelings, images, behaviours, appearance and life situation – clearly, in the moment, with a welcoming attitude of non-judgement and non-attachment. Self-love is the infusion of this inner acceptance with warmth, respect, understanding and compassion. The two – self-acceptance and self-love – create compassionate self-acceptance.

How compassionate self-acceptance leads to inner peace

At first glance the descriptions of self-acceptance and self-love sound like a recipe for passivism, for surely they preclude the need to change or improve? The reality is, however, that the process of compassionate self-acceptance often triggers deep changes that can cause us to evolve in ways we'd simply never have imagined possible. Rather than having our lives driven by resistance, fear and self-rejection, through compassionate self-acceptance we start to become driven by love, acceptance and self-expression. Your true self – not your ego – becomes in charge. The case study below demonstrates the difference.

CASE STUDY: DANIEL

Fifty-two-year-old Daniel was the managing director of a multi-million-pound company. Based on external appearances, he was a complete success. He owned three houses, drove an Aston Martin, wore designer clothes, had a beautiful wife and dined at the finest restaurants. He was driven, passionate and, with it, a very nice guy.

Daniel came to me because he was becoming increasingly aware of feeling dissatisfied with his life. He was no longer getting pleasure from holidays and going to nice places, and he was getting distracted at work. He knew something wasn't right and wanted some guidance as to what he could do to help himself. My first thought was that he might be depressed, but that turned out not to be the case. Gradually, it became apparent what was going on.

Daniel's feelings of being unsettled and dissatisfied were due to the conversation he was having with himself. I asked him to share with me a selection of his thoughts, which included: 'I should be richer', 'I should be able to help myself', 'I should have the answer', 'I need to try harder', 'I am useless'. It turned out that these thoughts had been with him most of his life and that he had dedicated a lot of his energy and time in trying to live up to them. However, as he had found out on many occasions, whatever he did and whatever he accomplished was not enough according to his thinking. What's more, he was aware that deep down inside him was a feeling of being flawed as a human being. His accomplishments (in his own words) were an attempt to hide these feelings of being bad.

My first priority with Daniel was to explain that what he was experiencing and feeling was very common and that he was, therefore, not alone in his predicament. The solution was not to try to improve himself (he had tried this without any lasting success), but to learn how to accept and love himself, just as he was. Daniel immediately shared the fear that a lot of people flag up, that if he accepted himself, he would not be motivated to change or improve his life. My answer to this was that the process of accepting yourself, just as you are, actually connects you to the internal resources and guidance which bring about change, not from a place of fear and limitation, but from a place of love and gratitude.

Within six months of starting the approach in this pillar, Daniel had turned his life around. He was much calmer and more accepting of himself (and others); he was able to enjoy and savour the fruits of his hard work; and, perhaps most importantly of all, he was now committed to being 'authentic' and honest in all of his relationships. Daniel was starting to find himself.

In each moment, you therefore have a choice. You can either choose the path of self-rejection (fighting against the reality of yourself as you are now) or choose the path of compassionate self-acceptance (the warm embrace of how you are in this moment). The gift in relating to yourself from compassionate self-acceptance, rather than self-rejection, is that a freedom, clarity, openness, sensitivity and joy start to arise spontaneously from within; you see intuitively what to do and how best to respond to your life situation. Rather than being driven by fear and self-rejection, your actions simply become an expression of who you truly are at the deepest level.

Why are self-acceptance and self-love important?

Self-acceptance and self-love are intrinsically connected to your levels of fulfilment, happiness and peace of mind. For example, people with high levels of self-acceptance and self-love:

- Are able to experience joy and freedom in most circumstances
- Feel the full spectrum of emotions without getting caught up in them
- Experience a deep connection to divinity, life, God or spirit
- Feel healthier, happier and more at peace
- Experience a deep gratitude and reverence for life
- Are present, awake and aware in the moment
- Are able to develop intimate and loving relationships with others
- Are better able to respond to life's challenges effectively and creatively

In my experience, someone with a high level of self-acceptance has an ease and lightness of being about them and an ability to accept life on life's terms. They have a natural reverence for life and a desire to protect the vulnerable and the environment. Society needs people who are more self-accepting!

How to accept and love yourself

There are many paths to self-acceptance and self-love, and the following approach is based on my own personal and professional experience of helping myself and others. Although this can be very challenging work, and requires a lot of courage and willingness, it has the potential to bring about profound changes in your emotional health and the way you feel and live your life.

The path to self-acceptance and self-love starts with a commitment to being more gentle and kind towards yourself. This means attending to the needs of your body and mind and relating to yourself in a way that honours your innate preciousness and value. Learning how to process your emotions (Pillar Two), heal grief (Pillar Six) and recover from trauma (Pillar Six) are important parts of this. It's about developing and deepening a loving relationship with yourself, while embracing your imperfections.

We are all perfectly imperfect human beings. We are all going to make 'mistakes', say the wrong things, berate ourselves, fail to meet our needs or upset people – and that's all OK; the key is to see that we are doing those things, learn from them, take responsibility for any consequences and move forwards – with renewed commitment to experiencing true happiness – to living with awareness, acceptance and integrity.

One of the best places to start your self-acceptance journey is with your body.

Make peace with your body

If you haven't done so already, I suggest you read my suggestions on meeting your physical needs (Pillar Four). Taking care of your body and nurturing it with healthy food, water, physical activity, sleep, rest and relaxation on an ongoing basis is for me at the heart of body acceptance.

In addition, I recommend that you put some time aside to do the following exercise. It takes about an hour or so. It's designed to explore and shift the relationship that you have to your body to one that is accepting and loving. It's a powerful exercise that I use in one of my workshops. If you think it might be too challenging to do this on your own, particularly if you have body-image issues, you might want to consider attending my workshop. Alternatively, you could do it in the presence of someone you trust and who is supportive of you.

EXERCISE: Make peace with your body

Here's what to do:

1. Write down all the different ways in which you don't accept your body. If you struggle with this, ask yourself: 'What would I change about my body if I could?' Don't hold back with your use of language! For example: 'I'm fat', I'm too short', 'I don't like my breasts; they are misshapen and ugly'.

2. Now write a list of what you do like about your body. If your instant response is, 'I don't like anything', take a couple of deep breaths and look in the mirror – you might find something. For example, 'I like my brown eyes', 'I like my long legs.'

3. Next, on a large piece of paper, draw a picture of your body – back and front; it doesn't have to be a work of art, just recognisable. Using different colours, shade in the areas that you don't love in a colour that feels appropriate. For each shaded area, write in the thought(s) you have about that part. Once that is completed, shade in the parts of you that you accept/like/love. This should be in a different colour – again, one that feels appropriate.

4. Having completed your drawing, focus on each body part in turn, starting with those that you don't like first:

   • Breathe deeply and allow yourself to locate where you are feeling the unprocessed emotional charge in your body. If you struggle with this, think back to an occasion when you were triggered by something and, as a result, started to think negatively about your body image.

- For each body part, process the emotional charge you are feeling using EmoTrance (page 53). Continue with each one, moving on to those parts you do like/love.

- If you sense any blocks to these, release them also, until you get to a stage when you look at the drawing of your body and not only don't feel any negativity but feel warmth towards your body. You may need to do this exercise a number of times but that's OK.

Let go of your resentments

One of the red-light warnings that you have yet to embrace emotional maturity is that you haven't fully processed the resentments that you carry. Letting go of resentments is a pre-requisite for compassionate self-acceptance.

Pretty much everyone has resentments, although not everyone realises it or will admit it. Resentments are bundles of toxic thoughts and emotions that stop you from thriving and flourishing. While unprocessed, they prevent you from being present, at peace and living with an open heart. I like to think of them as heavy emotional baggage or lead weights that we carry around with us; and it requires energy to not let go of them.

Most people who have experienced pain and hurt in relationship to someone or something else will have resentments. If someone burgled your house, or shouted at you, for example, after the initial shock, you would probably experience thoughts and feelings of resentment and anger. Deeper resentments happen when you have been deeply wounded (emotionally and physically). You might have been neglected in childhood or been attacked in adulthood – either can trigger the creation of that deadly bundle of thoughts and emotions. Although having resentments often feels uncomfortable, they can also provide a sense of righteousness, in that you feel justified in having them because of what happened. The problem, however, as I mentioned before, is that they are toxic to us.

The power of forgiveness

Forgiveness is the process by which you let go of your resentments. It's not about forgetting or minimising what has happened, but about reclaiming your energy so that you can live your life in a way that is no longer negatively influenced and limited by the issue about which you have resentment. Forgiveness is first and foremost for your benefit, not the other person's. Forgiveness is an act of self-love.

How to forgive

There are many different ways and processes involved in forgiveness. What follows is what I do with my patients (but see also Resources, page 291, for further reading).

Create a resentment inventory

You need to give yourself plenty of time to do this. Make a list of everyone and everything against which you have resentments, however minor. Remember, you have energy and life force trapped in that resentment, and this is your opportunity to reclaim it.

Once you have made your list, reorder it, so that the person or thing with which you have the strongest resentment is as the top. Watch out for your mind's tendency to gloss over someone. To know whether you have a resentment you need to slow down, breathe deeply and ask yourself, 'Do I hold any resentment against this person or thing?' Discomfort in your body suggests you do, although, of course, for some people and issues it will be obvious.

The principles with which I work the forgiveness process are as follows:

- Start getting the story clear about what exactly happened.

- Share that story with at least one person whom you trust and who can receive that story non-judgementally.

- Start processing the feelings that come up, especially anger and grief/sadness.

- Investigate your thoughts about that person using The Work (see Pillar One).

This might take an hour or a month. It may even take a couple of years if, for example, you were abused as a child, as it is quite normal and healthy to take time as you start to process the emotions around such an experience. You will know when it is complete when you truly feel at peace with that person. Unfortunately, the processing of your feelings is not something that happens automatically; it is something you need to take action on. There are many ways to process your emotions and Pillar Two has a number of suggestions. My preference is EmoTrance or Cradling.

You may or may not feel it is appropriate for you but for some patients, I take the work even deeper by asking them to research the life (or if that is not possible, to imagine the life) that the person has been living prior to the problem happening. The key is to get a real sense of what was going on for that person in that period of time. Your intention is to understand fully why they did what they did. For example, what was their childhood like (if you don't know, try to imagine)? What fears and insecurities were they operating from? How much shame and emotional pain were they in? To answer these, you might need to speak to relatives and friends, people who know this person. As you do this, more emotion will probably come up; as it does so, be gentle with yourself and process it, preferably in the presence of someone who can give you unconditional support. As you continue, compassion will eventually start to arise automatically.

The self-forgiveness process

One person not to forget about when it comes to resentments is yourself. Many people hold strong resentments against themselves because of something they have done or not done that they deemed unacceptable.

Andrew, a forty-year-old patient of mine, held three major resentments against himself. The first was that he never asked his childhood sweetheart to marry him (by the time he got round to doing it, she had found someone else). The second was that he hated the fact he was not richer and more successful. And the third was the time he hit his girlfriend (now wife). All three were restricting his ability to live a healthy, happy and fulfilling life.

For the first two, I got Andrew to follow the instructions for the for-giveness process. By allowing himself to feel his feelings fully and process them, after just one week he felt more at peace with himself. He also realised that the desire for wealth and fame was a belief he had borrowed from his father. For the third resentment, I encouraged him to make amends to his wife, then, having done so, to process any residual feeling.

Making amends

Making amends is the process of taking responsibility for your actions by communicating and apologising with sincerity and maturity to the person that you upset or hurt. Importantly, you then outline the actions you will take to make sure – as best you can – it doesn't happen again. Amends come from the heart, not the head. While Andrew had apologised 'a thousand times' and bought his wife many compensatory gifts, all of these words and actions were driven by guilt, not love. With his new insights Andrew was able to make amends to his wife. After he did so, they shared tears of sadness and relief with one another. Andrew remarked how he and his wife were feeling so much more alive, healthy and cleansed after this. That's the power of amends.

Experience self-love

For most people it is fairly easy to show kindness and love to others, but for most the real struggle and challenge is to experience uncondi-tional self-love. The following exercise is an adaptation of one I use in my workshop for you to use by yourself at home. I never cease to be amazed and humbled by the profound impact of this exercise on people's lives. If you find it difficult, I encourage you to come along to one of my workshops (see Resources, page 287). Alternatively, try the self-love meditation on page 223.

EXERCISE: The mirror

- Find a time when you will be completely alone and undisturbed for at least thirty minutes.

- Stand in front of a mirror – preferably a full-length one, and say to yourself out loud, while looking at yourself: 'I love you.' Don't worry if you don't mean it – this will still work!

- Do this again, but this time breathe deeply and slowly and say it slower: 'I – love – you.'

- As you say these words, become aware of your body. Where in your body do those words feel blocked? Where can you feel some discomfort? Most people feel it in their heart, stomach or throat area – but it can be anywhere. What you are feeling is just the trapped energy that is preventing these words from flowing through and energising your body.

- To release the block, silently tell the trapped energy to soften and flow – if it helps, massage the area gently. Eventually you will notice that the energy is moving. This can take a minute or two.

- Now sense which direction the energy wants to move in – it will be up, down, to the side, backwards or straight out of the body. The energy knows which way it wants to go!

- Now ask yourself, 'If this energy could exit my body, where would it choose to leave?' You should get a sense of it. The first time you do this, you'll be quite surprised because there will be a definite exit route – such as the top of the head, out the ears, eyes, mouth or nose, or maybe out of the hands or feet. Allow the energy to flow of your body, telling it gently and lovingly to 'soften and flow' as you go.

- Eventually, you'll sense that the energy has moved out of your body – this can take anywhere between a couple of seconds and twenty minutes – if it takes longer, just be patient, breathe deeply and 'soften and flow'. If you get to this stage, well done – you are doing really well!

- Now repeat the process, saying, 'I love you'. This time, the block might be in the same location or somewhere completely different.

Do exactly what you did before, until the energy has flowed out of the body completely. Then keep repeating until you get to the stage when saying the words, 'I love you' completely energises and uplifts you. When you feel those words, when you know in your heart that those words are true, then you have successfully completed this exercise.

EXERCISE: The self-love meditation

This is a powerful meditation that I used to use a lot in my early days of 'growing up'. Make sure you give yourself plenty of time for this and experience the way it positively shifts your energy and well-being.

- Sit still, close your eyes and take a couple of deep breaths in and out.

- Bring to mind someone or something for whom/which you have a deep unconditional love.

- If you can't think of anyone, imagine what the feelings would be like if you did have someone for whom you felt unconditional love.

- As you focus on that person or thing, notice what you are feeling in your body–mind and breathe in and out of those feelings, so that they start to expand.

- Once you can feel that loving appreciation in your body, release the image and send the loving appreciation that you are feeling down to your feet.

- Gradually move your attention up the entire length of your body, sending loving appreciation to every single cell. This might take a couple of seconds or minutes – do whatever feels comfortable or natural.

- Once you reach the top of your head, take some time to enjoy the peace and stillness. If you sense any blocks anywhere use Emo-Trance (page 53) to process it. Continue until your whole body is buzzing with warmth, expansion and self-love.

Discover and embrace your selves

If you're slightly perplexed by the title of the section, bear with me as this is one of the most important parts of this book. It builds on all the work you've done so far and is an essential part of accepting yourself.

The greatest personal and professional revelation for me in the last six years has been the discovery of the psychology of selves. Developed by two American psychologists, Hal and Sidra Stone, the theory of selves states that inside each of us is not just one personality but hundreds of sub-personalities, or selves. Each self is in effect a different person, with unique beliefs, perspectives, dislikes, likes, opinions, beliefs and feelings. However, we only identify with a handful of them – our so-called 'primary' selves. Some of the most common primary selves include the controlling self (this one is usually in charge of the other selves!), the inner critic, the perfectionist, the people pleaser, the protector, the responsible self, the sceptic, the joker, the serious self and the victim. Although you might think you are in charge, in reality your primary selves are in charge. You are, however, so much more than your primary selves – and this is where it gets really interesting.

The importance of embracing all your selves

What about those hundreds of other selves? These are the selves that for whatever reason we, over time, reject, deny, disown and push out of our awareness into our unconscious. Why do we reject these selves? Essentially, if any quality or trait belonging to a particular self was consistently suppressed by your caregivers you will reject that self in order to maintain a sense of connection to your caregivers (because they are the ones who ensure your survival). Furthermore, as you mould yourself to survive and manage your life situation during childhood, you will also reject the selves that are incompatible with the image that you have for yourself.

Some commonly disowned selves include the vulnerable child, the emotional self, the spiritual self, the fun self, the spontaneous self, the angry self, the damaged self, the rebel and the sensual self. You might think that not being in touch with some of these parts is actually a good thing – after all who wants to be angry, vulnerable or rebellious? Well there are three reasons why it's essential to get to know and embrace all of them. The first is that they each contain a gift for you. For example, the gift that comes with embracing our vulnerability is humility and a connection to our humanity. The gift that comes from embracing our rebelliousness can be creative self-expression and independent thought. The second reason is that by consciously getting in touch with these selves, you become in charge of them. Until you do this, they, to differing degrees, are in charge of you. The third and most important reason is because one of the master keys to true happiness is to accept and embrace all of the selves within us – no exceptions. This unconditional 'selves-acceptance' is what gives rise to the true self.

How to identify your disowned selves

So how do you start to become aware of your disowned selves? The first step is to write down a list of your primary selves and then think about and list their contrasting parts. So, for example, if you have a pusher self (a self that drives and pushes you hard) its opposite self will probably be the 'slob' or the 'easy-going' self. If you strongly identify with your 'intellectual' self, your disowned self will probably be the 'emotional' or the 'vulnerable' self.

Another very good way to identify your disowned selves is by observing those moments when you are strongly judgemental, critical or overly admiring of another person. For example, a disowned self of mine was the angry self, and until a couple of years ago I wasn't aware of this – I'd just assumed that I was calm most of the time. However, the clue that I had rejected my anger lay in the fact that I was extremely uncomfortable around and judgemental of others who were angry. By using voice dialogue, a process that allows you to speak with your different selves, I was able to understand and embrace that angry part of me. In doing so I was able to access its gifts – power, strength and assertiveness. What's more, I no longer over-react to angry people. So embracing my angry self (and other disowned selves) has been a real blessing for me. Doing this work has also been transformative for many of the patients and students I have taught it to.

I strongly encourage you to take some time to identify your various selves. All selves want to be acknowledged, accepted and understood. If you are committed to true happiness and compassionate self-acceptance, this is a really important task.

The exercise below is a great way of doing this. It uses the voice dialogue process developed by Hal and Sidra Stone. It's a simple way to get to know each of your selves and, in doing so, reclaim all of the parts that you have disowned or ignored. The exercise does require a partner. However, it is very easy to do and a vital element of the experience is that it's light-hearted so you can reassure your partner or friend that they're not required to play the part of a psychologist! In fact it often helps if you play the part of the facilitator first. The only rule for the facilitator is that they be accepting, understanding and non-judgemental of the selves they speak to.

Do give the exercise plenty of time. While it is safe and very easy to do, if you are unsure about it, take a look at my website www.discovertruehappiness.com, which has a video of me demonstrating the process.

EXERCISE: How to meet your selves

Let's assume that you are going to be the facilitator and that you are going to speak to the selves in your partner or friend.

- Sit opposite your partner, take a couple of deep breaths and say to your partner 'I would like to speak to the controlling self.' (I tend to start with the controlling self, because this is the one that is in charge.)

- Your partner should immediately respond with the words 'I am the controlling self.' You can then start talking to their controlling self. Your partner should speak as the controlling self – this will happen automatically, he/she doesn't have to do anything to make it happen. Just trust and it will happen. No thinking and no effort is required.

- As the facilitator your job is to ask the self you are speaking to some questions. Your intention at this stage is simply to get to know it and learn about it. For example: What is your job? How long have you known XX for? (Substitute XX with your partner's name.) How important are you to XX? How have you protected XX? What's the one thing XXX needs to hear, know or experience right now? Having done this, I suggest you then ask their controlling self the following 'I am now going to speak to another self, would you be willing to prevent any self other than the one I want to speak with from interrupting?'. 'Would you also be prepared to stop yourself from interrupting?' Because the controlling self's nature is to control, it almost always responds with 'yes'. This helps to prevent interference from other selves such as the sceptic, fear or the controller itself. You are now free to engage other selves. You might, for example, want to explore the rational self, and then the emotional self.

Once you and your partner have both finished using voice dialogue take some time to reflect on the experience. It can be life changing – I'm not saying that lightly. Most people are amazed to meet certain parts of themselves and to gain some understanding of how that self has influenced their life. The experience allows you to really gain an understanding of why you are the way you are.

CASE STUDY: JAMES

James was a successful businessman who came to see me partly because he was struggling to be emotionally intimate with his partner. Like many men, he found it difficult to get in touch with and accept his more sensitive, vulnerable side. It may seem surprising but using voice dialogue is such cases is very appropriate – successful businessmen, though sometimes a little sceptical initially, quickly appreciate the efficiency and effectiveness of the process.

When I did the voice dialogue exercise with James it soon became apparent that his controlling self was protecting his scared and lonely four-year-old self. Having uncovered this, I asked to speak to the loving and very caring part of him (the compassionate self) and asked if it was willing to take care of the vulnerable child – also, if it sensed any block to doing that. The answer was yes, it would love to take care of the vulnerable child but there was a block – in the form of the twelve-year-old part of James, who felt fed-up and ignored.

When such blocks emerge it's important that they are acknowledged and the rejected 'self' is accepted: in this case, the twelve-year-old part of James needed to feel loved and taken care of too. This can be achieved through a short exercise where the 'rejected' self accepts the loving energy of their caring self and that that energy will be now be a constant presence. (You can view the video of me demonstrating the process in the voice dialogue section of my website www.drmarkatkinson.com.)

Once James had completed his session, I asked how he felt. His response was 'very balanced, present'. He was also aware of a sense of well-being. When I asked him to tune into his twelve- and four-year-old parts, he commented on how much warmth and care he was feeling. The key to the transformation was not just accessing these parts, but facilitating the care of the young parts by the compassionate self. A month later he told me he felt so much at peace with himself and that he found it much easier to share his thoughts and feelings with his partner. His partner was apparently delighted. This is the power of voice dialogue.

The value of knowing your selves

What we are doing through voice dialogue is getting to know and accept ourself or, more accurately, our selves. What's more, by working with opposing energies of two opposite selves a third energy naturally emerges, called the aware ego. This is very important. Accessing the aware ego enables you to experience the energy of two opposite selves – for example, the rational self and the emotional self – in a way that is healthy and balanced.

So, by accessing your aware ego you are able to access and draw upon these energies when you want to, depending on the situation you are in. When you are identified with one of the selves, to the exclusion of its opposite self, your ability to respond to a situation is limited. Take relationships, for example: the rational self is not the ideal self to build intimacy, neither is being over-identified with the emotional self – you need a balance between the two. That's what you get having explored these two selves. So, rather than being limited by any of these selves, you are now able to use them to empower you in your life, relationship and career.

TAKING VOICE DIALOGUE FURTHER

In addition to the selves or voices explored above, there are also many other voices that can be accessed or awakened using voice dialogue. These transcendental, or non-dualistic, voices are related to higher spiritual functions and include the middle way, deep appreciation, no-mind, feminine compassion, pure joy, and so on. Many people spend years in meditation practice trying to experience them, and while this most definitely has its role to play, you can access them instantly using voice dialogue. Dennis Genpo Merzel has pioneered this application of voice dialogue. If you're intrigued by voice dialogue, take a look at his work (see Resources, page 287).

Awaken to the true self

The culmination of my work with voice dialogue has been to use it to access the true self that I first mentioned in Pillar One. To re-iterate, the true self:

- Knows how to get in touch with and realise our fullest potential

- Is experienced as a deep sense of well-being, vitality and peace of mind

- Knows the perfect response to each unfolding moment

- Is the source of creativity and intuition

- Provides us with clarity, insight, guidance and natural confidence

By working on the pillars in this book you will inevitably move towards finding your true self. However, the use of voice dialogue can really help accelerate that process. The reason for this is that it helps you 'get past' your dualistic selves, i.e. those opposing selves such as your rational self and your emotional self, and access your non-dualistic true self.

This might seem like pretty advanced stuff but often it's simply the language that people find a little awkward. Just trust the process and give the exercise below a go. You will need to do this with a partner or as part of a group (you can find details of such groups on the website www.discovertruehappiness.com). It may feel a little strange doing this exercise at first, but if you approach it in a relaxed, light-hearted manner – and take your time over it – you'll soon begin to get the hang of it.

EXERCISE: Accessing the true self with voice dialogue

- Relax somewhere quiet, where you won't be disturbed.

- Your partner should say to you 'I would like to speak to the dualistic self'. Take a moment to allow the energy of the dualistic self to arise (you will feel quite different). When it does, respond with 'I am the dualistic self'. Then share what it is like to be the dualistic self. Your partner can ask various questions such as how does it feel to be the dualistic self? Please tell me about yourself? What do you want for XX (whatever your name is)?

- Having done this, your partner should then ask 'I would like to speak to the non-dual self'. You should then affirm that you are the non-dual self. Your partner can ask questions such as who are you, or who are you not? The latter is more appropriate for the non-dual self!

- Once that is complete, your partner should say to you, 'now I would like to speak to the true self, the self that includes, yet transcends the dualistic self and the non-dual self.' Affirm yourself as the true self and, as before, your partner can ask various questions such as how does it feel to be the true self? Please tell me about yourself? What do you want for XX? What does XX need to do in order to fully embrace you? Having finished, reflect on what has emerged.

This exercise is truly important for a number of reasons. Firstly, you will experience a deep sense of peace, well-being and balance when you are 'in' the true self. This not only feels great, but it gives you a feeling of freedom that many people have never experienced. Secondly, the true self knows the perfect response to everything, so allowing it to make suggestions can be very enlightening.

ACCESSING THE TRUE SELF WITH THE GATEWAY

The gateway is a psycho-spiritual tool that I have developed for welcoming and integrating all of the selves that are creating blocks and barriers to true happiness. At the heart of the gateway is the discovery that these 'selves' have a tangible presence in the physical body, and that by enquiring as to what they want at the deepest level they will lead you into the direct experience of the true self. By then re-integrating that self into the true self, its hidden gifts and energy become fully liberated. The revelation revealed through the gateway is that all of the aspects of ourselves that we relate to in a negative light are actually gateways into higher states of consciousness and our true self. All we have to do is welcome these parts and enquire into their deepest intention for us. It is a profound process that I use with most of my patients and on my workshops. I'd love you to try. Instructions for it can be found on my website www.discovertruehappiness.com.

Living as your true self

While voice dialogue – and the gateway – can help you get in touch with and experience the true self, to access it and live as the true self most of the time is no easy task. It requires work and commitment. So, what work exactly? Well, you've been doing it all along – the path to the true self involves growing up, waking up and living with HEART (Honesty, Emotional Awareness, Authenticity, Responsibility and Trust).

PILLAR SEVEN: Summary

- Lack of self-acceptance and self-love is a major cause of unhappiness, mental ill health and life dissatisfaction.

- Self-acceptance is the process of bringing an inner acceptance to the reality, right now, of every part of you – warts and all. Self-love is the infusion of this inner acceptance with warmth, respect, understanding and compassion.

- Resentments are toxic bundles of thoughts and feelings that prevent you from knowing inner peace and self-love.

- You are made up of hundreds of different selves. Through using voice dialogue you can start to discover and embrace them all – this leads to a deep sense of self-understanding and self-acceptance.

- The true self is that aspect of our being that includes and yet transcends all of our dualistic selves. The true self is the source of true happiness.

- The path to the true self involves growing up, waking up and living with HEART.

Pillar Eight: Create positive, healthy relationships

One of our deepest needs is to belong – to feel connected to others and to have positive, healthy relationships.[100] Open, honest relationships in which we are truly accepted for what we are (not necessarily for what we do) are a tonic for the soul and a key contributor to our emotional health and happiness. Indeed one study reported in the *British Medical Journal* found that the only difference between the top 10 per cent of happiest people and everyone else is their rich and satisfying social lives. [101]

We all need relationships. We are social creatures designed to be in relationship to others. Years ago, our family would have consisted of mum, dad, uncles, aunts, grandparents and trusted friends, all of whom played an active role in bringing us up. But in some parts of the Western world, the social unit has been reduced to a handful of often self-centred individuals. More and more people are feeling isolated, fearful of the community they live within and caught up in the circumstances of their life.

CASE STUDY: GLORIA

Gloria was a successful forty-something executive who, despite living a pretty lavish lifestyle and being the life and soul of the party, was feeling 'disconnected and numb on the inside'. Having had numerous short-term relationships, all of which turned sour within a couple of months, she had now found the man of her dreams, but was terrified of losing him because of her track record of 'relationship failure'. What's more, Gloria didn't have any true friends – plenty of so-called acquaintances, but no one with whom she was able to share her inner life.

After some time and exploration, it turned out that Gloria had undiagnosed depression and a history of physical and emotional abuse, which had never been addressed. Furthermore, she had never developed the necessary skills to make her friendships and intimate relationships work. She had assumed that relationships took care of themselves.

My work with Gloria spanned a period of six months, in which time we addressed her depression and trauma and I taught her some of the friendship and intimate relationship-nourishing skills from this pillar. Her progress was initially slow, but she gradually started investing time in her relationships and doing the necessary work. Within six months, she had two close friends and her relationship with her partner was starting to flourish. By being open and honest and willing to process the emotions that came up for her as she went along, she not only started to feel more connected than at any other time in her life, but her depression had lifted and, in doing so, had revealed a sensitive, loving side to her. Gloria was starting to discover her true self through her relationships.

What is a positive, healthy relationship?

This type of relationship is life-affirming and is based on openness, honesty and mutual respect. The bond that is created involves understanding and support and is associated with feelings of warmth, care and connectedness. The key to a positive relationship is for each person to relate to the other as an equal. Of course, it's not realistic for these qualities to exist all of the time, but within a relationship, whether a friendship or a couple, they should be present more often than not.

One of the keys to developing positive, healthy relationships is to realise that they require time, patience, effort and persistence; they rarely happen naturally.

In contrast to positive relationships are toxic relationships. These are predominantly based on defensiveness, dishonesty, disrespect and lack of, or absence of, meaningful emotional contact. While toxic relationships might look OK on the outside, they drain your energy and prevent you from fulfilling your potential and creating a healthy and fulfilling life.

The following are defined behaviours within relationships that can both contribute to and help grow a relationship, or destroy intimacy, trust and connection.[102]

Positive and healthy	Toxic and unhealthy
Appreciation	Criticism
Positive attention	Negative attention
Listening	Ignoring/interrupting
Joking	Character assassinations
Intimacy	Withholding
Fun	Lack of fun
Respect	Disrespect
Keeping promises	Breaking promises
Compromising	Refusing to compromise
Supporting	Ridiculing
Encouraging	Putting down
Treating as equals	Parenting
Complimenting	Insincerity
Offering advice	Forcing unwanted advice
Confronting	Attacking
Facing reality	Denial or avoidance of reality
Being open	Being defensive
Flexibility	Rigidity
Authenticity	Lack of honesty
Turning towards your partner during stress	Turning away
Solving problems together	Solving problems separately
Giving/receiving love	Being closed to love
Balanced closeness/separateness	Separateness/enmeshed
Appreciating their differences	Resisting their differences

Many of us will unknowingly be using a whole bunch of toxic behaviours – why? Because we aren't aware that they are toxic and because we aren't aware of what healthy relationships look like. The suggestions offered in this pillar will show you how to change that and create positive, healthy relationships.

How positive, healthy relationships benefit your health

Fulfilling your basic human desire for connection and experiencing intimacy through partners, friendships, groups, community, animals and nature are essential for deep healing and happiness.

By way of illustration, a 1992 study reported in the *American Journal of Epidemiology* provided an interesting insight into the correlation between love and physical health. For a five-year period, a university research project studied 8500 men who had no previous history or symptoms of ulcers. By the end of the study 250 of the men had developed ulcers. What was the variable? Those men who reported a low level of love from their wives were more than twice as likely to have ulcers as those who reported a high level. [103]

The power of friendship

An important contributor to a healthy, meaningful and fulfilling life is friends. We all know this instinctively – friends provide warmth, laughter, shared experiences, a sympathetic ear, support – but you may be surprised just how vitally important they are. One Australian study found that maintaining friendships was even more important than family when it came to living a longer life. Over 1500 people aged seventy plus were asked about their level of contact with friends, relatives and children. Their health was then monitored over a ten-year period. While contact with their children or relatives didn't have an appreciable impact on how long they lived, contact with their network of friends did.[104] Another study found that people who feel isolated are three to five times more likely to die prematurely and get sick than those who don't.[105]

So what is a friend? According to the *Concise Oxford English Dictionary* a friend is: 'One joined to another in intimacy and mutual benevolence independently of sexual or family love; a person who acts for one; sympathiser; helper; patron; one who is not an enemy; one who is on the same side.' Put another way, a friend is someone you know, like, respect and trust. Taking time to develop and deepen your friendships is a powerful contributor to your happiness. Self-disclosure – the sharing of thoughts, feelings and facts about oneself and one's life situation – that is reciprocated is one of the most important keys to friendship building.[106]

So let's get practical and look at how you can begin to improve your relationships. It's not an overstatement to say that positive, healthy relationships can transform your life!

Practise empathy and loving-kindness

Think back to a moment when you felt completely heard, accepted and understood by another person, a moment when you felt connected to them and safe. This is the experience of empathy, and creating empathy is a key skill for anyone who is committed to waking up, growing up and becoming truly happy.

How to practise empathy

Empathy, for me, involves being fully present to another person with our whole being and allowing oneself to fall into harmony and resonance with them. You are not evaluating or judging them – just deeply hearing and receiving them as they are. Being in a state of empathy allows you to get a sense of their world, without losing your own authentic sense of self. It's not about agreeing with that person but demonstrating that you understand them and that you are willing to enter their world. You know you are in an empathic connection with someone when you feel a sense of aliveness and connection between you both. When someone has been empathic with you, you will feel understood, you'll probably experience a release of tension and the need to speak will evaporate. Empathy is, of course, a vital skill for developing positive, healthy relationships.

Tips for developing empathy

Most of us are so caught up in our own thoughts and issues that we rarely have the presence or time to attend deeply to the experience of another person. What's more, unless we learn how to manage our thoughts and emotions and come to a level of compassionate self-acceptance, it's harder to truly be there for someone else. But like much of what I have shared so far, it's a skill that can be learnt and one that gets easier the more you practise it.

Make connection a priority

One way to transform and enrich your personal relationships is to make connection a priority whenever you've spent time away from your partner. The rule is, therefore, that when you come together, you don't talk about problems or the day you had – you immediately come together, hug/kiss and say, for example, 'I've missed you' and exchange small talk for a few minutes. This is about reconnecting and falling into harmony with one another, following which you can then each do what you need to do. This process of connection is a real tonic for relationships.

Practise empathic listening

Next time someone starts speaking to you, take a couple of slow breaths and give your full attention to them with the intention of hearing and truly understanding what they are saying and where they are coming from. Avoid the temptation to think about what they are saying; just listen. Once they have finished, paraphrase what you have heard them say and feed that back to them. This is empathic listening and is at the heart of respectful communication. If empathy is a challenge for you, as it was for me, I highly recommend an empathy training course based on the principles of an enlightened approach to communication, called Non-violent Communication (see Resources, page 291).

Enter their world

Think of someone you don't like. Now take five minutes to imagine that you are that person. Close your eyes and imagine you have lived their entire life and are living it now. Avoid the tendency to judge, hold an intention to understand truly why they are the way they are. Trust your imagination in presenting to you images and a sense of what has happened to them in their lifetime. Really allow yourself to get a feel for what it must be like to be them. Once you have finished this process, imagine that they are now in front of you – notice how different you feel towards them.

Stay open and positive

A sure way to kill empathy is to shoot down someone else's perspective or opinion, patronise, disagree routinely, interrupt frequently, change the subject, give unwanted advice, criticise, be insincere, withhold your truth, use sarcasm or play games/manipulate others. There are, of course, many other toxic behaviours (see the introductory section to this pillar, page 235). If you tend to use one or more of these, next time you start to use them, switch to being open and positive, either by acknowledging what the other person has said (empathic listening) or saying something positive in a way that is sincere. Changing toxic behaviours to nourishing ones takes time and patience, but it's an essential component of creating empathy.

Practise loving-kindness

The exercise below is one of my favourite meditations and one that can help you open your heart and create and deepen loving relationships with others. A 2008 study found that people who practised loving-kindness on a daily basis experienced an increase in emotions, such as love, joy, gratitude, contentment and hope; they also benefited from an increase in mindfulness, self-acceptance, positive relationships and good physical health, as well as increased life satisfaction.[107]

EXERCISE: Loving-kindness meditation

There is a variety of different approaches to loving-kindness, but this exercise is the one that I use successfully with many of my patients. You might want to start by reading through the instructions a couple of times, so that you can then do this with your eyes closed. (Alternatively, you could follow the instructions on a guided meditation CD – see Resources, page 285).

- Find a quiet, comfortable place where you won't be disturbed for at least fifteen minutes.

- Bring to mind someone or something for whom/which you have a deep unconditional love. If you can't think of anyone, imagine what the feelings would be like if you did have someone for whom you felt unconditional love.

- Allow those feelings to build up within you, especially around the area of the heart.

- Now gently allow the loving-kindness to flow into every part of your body. Include any sensations that might feel uncomfortable. Continue until your body is full of the energy of love and appreciation.

- Now turn your attention to any thoughts, feelings and images you might have. Send that loving energy to all of them, welcome each and every one of them as equals; be unconditional in your sharing of your love. Breathe deeply and allow this process to happen.

- If your mind wanders or if you feel tense, return your attention to your breath and continue following the instructions with a lightness and gentleness.

- Now turn your attention to the whole of your body–mind. Again, with gentleness, allow loving-kindness to envelop and permeate your body–mind; allow yourself to experience and enjoy the preciousness of this moment.

- Now visualise or sense someone close to you who is suffering. On your next in-breath take in this person's suffering – allow their dark energy of suffering to ride the in-breath into your heart where it will dissolve completely. Don't worry about taking on board their energy; the heart will dissolve it fully.

- On the out-breath, breathe out loving-kindness to that person; see it entering them.

- Now keep repeating the in-breath and out-breath for a few minutes, as described above. Then ask yourself is there anything you can do to help and support them? Allow an answer to come.

- Now imagine all of your family and friends standing or sitting in front of you. Breathe in their suffering and allow it to dissolve in your heart. Now allow loving-kindness to emanate out of you (on the out-breath) and flow into them. Continue for a few minutes.

- Now imagine a group comprising all the people you don't like or don't get on well with. Breathe in their suffering and allow it to dissolve in your heart. Now allow loving-kindness to emanate out of you (on the out-breath) and flow into them. Continue for a few minutes.

- Now imagine all living beings; you can include the natural world as well. Breathe in their suffering and allow it to dissolve in your heart. Now allow loving-kindness to emanate out of you (on the out-breath) and flow into them. Continue for a few minutes.

- Once you have finished, take a minute or two to enjoy what you are feeling and to notice how your heart has softened.

When you first try this meditation, it might feel false or uncomfortable, particularly if you aren't used to doing anything like this. My advice is to persist with it, despite those feelings and thoughts, and within a couple of sessions (based on my experience with patients), you should start to notice a real shift in the way you feel and relate to others. Obviously, you can use it as often or as infrequently as you want, but I'd recommend that for the first few weeks you try to do it most days.

Practise the four As of healthy, mature relationships

There are four different practices, in addition to empathy, that I regard as being essential to healthy mature relationships. They are attention, acceptance, appreciation and affection. As water is to life, these four are to healthy relationships.

Attention

What is it like when someone provides you with their whole undivided attention? It might be unnerving if you've rarely experienced it before, however for most people, being with someone who is truly present, available and focused on them to the exclusion of all other distractions is a dream come true, particularly if that person embodies the other three As! Paying attention to another person with the intention of truly listening to and hearing what they have to say provides the foundations for intimacy and connection. Here's how you can cultivate attention:

- Over the next twenty-four hours, whenever your partner speaks to you, give them your full, undivided attention. Make sure your body is turned towards them. Breathe deeply and relax any tension in your body; allow it to be as natural as possible.

- Plan quality time together. It's easy to get absorbed in work, TV and other activities. Make an effort to share your thoughts and feelings with your partner (and to receive theirs) on most days. It just takes ten to fifteen minutes. Plan date nights (and keep them); choose fun things to do together.

- Incorporate the remaining As when you do this.

Acceptance

In Pillar Seven I examined compassionate self-acceptance, a way of responding to yourself that is both loving and accepting. This is not only essential in order to reduce the power of negative thoughts and self-criticism, but also in order to thrive and flourish. Applying the same principles to others, especially your partners and friends, is one of the keys to cultivating intimacy and understanding.

Have you ever had the experience of being truly accepted by another person? Can you recall how you felt in response to it? Being allowed to be who you are – with all of your feelings, opinions, insecurities, fears and choices – allows you to feel safe, and that safety is the essential ingredient in healthy, loving relationships. By accepting someone as they are, you are honouring their right to have the feelings and thoughts they are having. As long as they are not being abusive to you or crossing certain boundaries, giving someone the space to be themselves in their entirety is not only an enlightening experience for them but also an empowering and healing experience for you. When you accept someone, you are sending a message to them, at a deep level, that they are OK as they are.

Tips for learning acceptance

Resist the urge to control

Next time you are with your partner notice any urge to control them. When you become aware of the urge arising, note where you feel it in your body and breathe into it. You could use EmoTrance to process what you are feeling (see page 53).

Adjust your expectations

For a day, drop all expectations of your partner, and notice how this changes the way you relate to them and how your stress levels reduce considerably.

Use your breathing

Next time you are talking to your partner, while paying attention to them, focus on your breathing; breathe deeply and do your best to allow them to be as they are (unless they are being abusive towards you). If it helps, imagine them in a bubble within which are contained all of their emotions, fears, beliefs and opinions. This will help you to be less affected by the way you are. As you get better at this you can drop the bubble.

Appreciation

Once attention is in place, sharing genuine and sincere appreciation with the person you are with is one of the quickest and most effective ways to open the floodgates of connection. Studies consistently show that if the ratio of positive feelings and interactions to negative ones is above 5:1, the likelihood of creating and sustaining a healthy, intimate relationship is increased considerably.[108] Here are a couple of suggestions to help you with this.

Make an appreciation list

Write down a list of all the things that you appreciate about your partner. If you get stuck, try to recall what first drew you to them. Having written the list, share one of the things on it with your partner each day for the next seven days. You will probably feel awkward doing this to begin with and it might feel false, but most people relax into it very quickly. The idea, when sharing appreciations, is to be as sincere as possible. If you feel tense about this, remember to breathe deeply.

Share appreciations

As you get better at delivering appreciations, start noticing spontaneous moments and opportunities to share them. Don't go overboard – you do need to find a balance here – but as you go through your day, offer random acts or remarks of appreciation to people you meet: 'You look well', 'It's really good to see you' and so on. Keep them short, to the point, relevant and, most important of all, genuine.

Affection

Affectionate behaviour is any behaviour that is genuinely intended to convey care, respect, appreciation and love. It can be verbal (for example, 'I love you'), non-verbal (kisses, hugs and holding hands) or it could be expressed through providing support or taking action in order to help another person. At the heart of the affection is sincerity and the absence of any self-motive or self-interest. Like attention, acceptance and appreciation, regular experiences of affection help considerably to develop the depth of your emotional bond.

How much affectionate behaviour is there between you and your partner? To answer this, score yourself between zero (= none whatsoever) and ten (= very affectionate). If you score less than eight read on:

- Both you and your partner should write down what you consider affectionate behaviours to be and ways in which the other could be more affectionate.

- Talk openly with your partner about affection, what it means to you and decide how you can increase your levels of affection – for example holding hands more, hugging a couple of times a day, giving/receiving a massage in the evening, more affectionate lovemaking.

- If you and/or your partner are fearful of affection, you should explore the reasons why this is so. Doing this work with a therapist might help.

- Sexual intimacy is built on the foundations for emotional and physical intimacy. If you and your partner are having any problems relating to sexual intimacy, see Resources, page 291, for recommended reading.

Identify the presence of co-dependency or counter-dependency

One of the most common barriers to experiencing emotional health and healthy relationships is co-dependency and counter-dependency. At least 95 per cent of the people who come to me with emotional-health problems and/or addictions have patterns of emotionally immature behaviours, attitudes and emotional-management styles that are limiting their progression into emotional maturity and their ability to experience healthy intimacy. For example, a considerable number of the people I work with tend to blame others for their problems and/or avoid reality and their 'uncomfortable' emotions at all costs. While it's tempting to think or 'joke' that it's just down to having not 'emotionally grown up', clinicians and researchers have discovered that these are actually symptoms of a failure to complete two of the most important developmental processes of childhood: emotional bonding and psychological separation.[109]

Deep, secure bonding with caregivers provides the foundations upon which emotional health, happiness and self-esteem are built.[110] If your parents were able to reliably and consistently provide the cuddles, positive affirmation and emotional nurturing and responsiveness that you needed, a strong emotional bond between you and them is created. This provides the necessary internal sense of trust, safety and security that enables you to explore the outside world and, in doing so, start the process of emotionally and psychologically separating from your parents.

By the age of three, and given the right conditions, most children should have completed their second 'birth' – the 'psychological' birth. Having done this, they will have a healthy and positive sense of self, be able to regulate their feelings and behaviour, experience self-confidence and be able to engage with others co-operatively and as equals. If, however, this natural process is interfered with or blocked, two patterns of behaviour and relating will emerge, depending on when and how the interference took place. The two limiting patterns are called co-dependency and counter-dependency.

Co-dependency

Co-dependency is a pattern of dependency, neediness and low self-esteem that is caused primarily by traumatic bonding breaks within the first six months of life. Being separated from their mother, physically neglected or having a mother who wasn't sensitively attuned and responsive to their needs and cues are just some of the experiences that could result in a child subsequently developing a co-dependency pattern of behaviours.

Counter-dependency

Counter-dependency behaviours result when psychological separation fails to take place because of emotional, physical and/or sexual abuse or neglect. Emotional abuse occurs any time a parent interacts with their child in a way that undermines their emotional development – this includes denial of affection, using the child to meet their own emotional needs, criticising, humiliating the child, verbally abusing the child and so on. What constitutes physical and sexual abuse is more obvious, but bear in mind that it includes what may seem to be more minor acts such as pinching and shaking. Neglect is the persistent lack of appropriate care, including love, stimulation, safety, nourishment, warmth, education and medical attention.

Unlike people with co-dependent behaviour patterns, who tend to come across as needy, weak and insecure, individuals with counter-dependent behaviours cover up their neediness and low self-esteem by projecting an aura of calm, confidence and strength.

How co-dependent and counter-dependent behaviours differ

The following chart from the book *The Flight from Intimacy* (see Resources, page 291) highlights the behavioural differences between someone with co-dependency and counter-dependency. It is normal to shift between the two sets of behaviours at different times.

Co-dependent behaviours	Counter-dependent behaviours
Clings to others	Pushes others away
Acts weak and vulnerable	Acts strong and invulnerable
Is overwhelmed by his/her feelings	Is cut off from his/her feelings
Is other-centred	Is self-centred
Is addicted to people	Is addicted to activities and substances
Is easily invaded by others	Is 'armoured' against others' attempts to get close
Has low self-esteem	Has falsely inflated self-esteem
Acts incompetent	Tries to 'look good'
Has depressed energy	Has manic energy
Acts insecure	Acts secure
Acts weak	Acts strong
Feels guilty	Blames others
Craves intimacy and closeness	Avoids intimacy and closeness
Acts self-effacing	Acts grandiose
Has victim behaviours	Tries to victimise others first
Is a people pleaser	Is a people-controller
Suffered neglect as a child	Suffered abuse as a child

While it is normal to have features of both co- and counter-dependency, if you look back over your lifetime, one or other pattern will usually stand out as being dominant. The good news is that you can become free from these patterns of behaviour by completing the uncompleted process of bonding and separation yourself by following my suggestions.

Are you co-dependent or counter-dependent?

Go through the questionnaires below to establish which way you are leaning. Score each question as follows:

No = 0, Occasionally = 1, Yes = 2

QUESTIONNAIRE: Co-dependency

Do you:

- Worry that other people will reject you? ☐

- Tend to assume responsibility for other people's feelings and/or behaviours? ☐

- Find it hard to trust yourself and/or make decisions? ☐

- Experience repeated emotional crises and chaos in your life? ☐

- Try to please others through what you say and do? ☐

- Have few or more physical, emotional or intellectual boundaries? ☐

- Get overwhelmed by your feelings? ☐

- Have perfectionist tendencies? ☐

- Judge yourself harshly? ☐

- Have a tendency to experience guilt? ☐

- Tend to feel victimised or act like a martyr? ☐

- Tend to take care of the needs of others, rather than yourself? ☐

- Feel anxious and insecure without knowing why? ☐

- Tend to value other people's opinions more than your own? ☐

- Need to be in relationships in which you feel needed? ☐

Total score ☐

QUESTIONNAIRE: Counter-dependency

Do you:

- Have a strong need to be right? ☐

- Need to look successful, secure and competent? ☐

- Rarely allow yourself to be vulnerable or weak? ☐

- Find it hard to be aware of your feelings? ☐

- Have difficulty relaxing and doing nothing? ☐

- Rarely ask others to meet your needs and wants? ☐

- Struggle to be intimate with another person? ☐

- Get bored easily and seek new thrills? ☐

- Feel that you are entitled to special treatment by others? ☐

- Dislike asking for help? ☐

- Feel a strong need to have all of the right answers? ☐

- Struggle to know what you need or want? ☐

- Find it hard to admit mistakes or to apologise? ☐

- Fear being controlled or smothered by other people? ☐

- Have a tendency to deny, discount or underplay the problems in your life? ☐

Total score ☐

Addressing co- or counter-dependent behaviour

If you scored 12 or more on either questionnaire you will benefit from taking the steps outlined below. I also strongly recommend you read the books on co-dependency and counter-dependency that I mention in the Resources section, page 291, in particular the work of Barry and Janae Weinhold.)

For mainly co-dependent behaviours

If you have mainly co-dependent behaviours, I recommend you focus on and address the following:

- Increasing your autonomy and becoming more independent (see the emotional needs section in Pillar Three)

- Identifying and addressing any underlying addictions and trauma (Pillar Six)

- Learning how to cope and manage strong feelings (Pillars One and Two)

- Developing compassionate self-acceptance (Pillar Seven)

- Building and maintaining boundaries (Pillar Eight)

- Identifying and living from your highest values (Pillar Three)

- Learning how to develop healthy, mature relationships (Pillar Eight)

For mainly counter-dependent behaviours

If you have mainly counter-dependent behaviours, I recommend you focus on and address the following:

- Identifying and addressing any underlying addictions and trauma (Pillar Six)

- Enhancing your emotional awareness and emotional literacy (Pillar Two)

- Developing the skills of intimacy and empathy (Pillar Eight)

- Developing compassion for others and yourself (Pillar Seven)

- Replacing 'walls' with flexible healthy boundaries (Pillar Eight)

- Improving listening skills (Pillar Eight)

- Embracing your vulnerable selves (Pillar Seven)

- Learning how to develop healthy, mature relationships (Pillar Eight)

Consider working with a professional

Although you can make significant improvements by following my own advice, if you feel your symptoms are serious, you may benefit immensely from working with a therapist who is familiar with co-dependency and counter-dependency (see Resources, page 288).

One of the best ways to move from co-dependency and counter-dependency into emotional maturity is, with the guidance of a therapist, for you and your partner (if you have one) to commit to helping each other do this work. As a general rule, people with co-dependent behaviours tend to choose life partners with counter-dependent behaviours.

Consider a treatment programme or workshop

If your symptoms of co-dependency or counter-dependency are severe, impairing your ability to live a healthy and functional life, or causing problems with addictions or your relationships, you might want to consider going into a co-dependency treatment programme or attending a specialist workshop (see Resources, page 288).

Support groups

If you are a co-dependent or counter-dependent you might benefit from attending Co-dependents Anonymous (CODA), a support group and fellowship of men and women who are committed to creating healthy and intimate relationships through sharing their experience, strength and hope (see Resources, page 288).

Develop and maintain healthy boundaries

One of the key skills to master when creating positive, healthy relationships is that of boundaries. A boundary is an invisible fence or space that you put in place in order to protect yourself and maintain your sense of self without offending others. They also alert you to when others are intruding. A boundary is made up of your sense of worth, your identity, your rights and your right to express and defend those rights. Boundaries are an essential ingredient in all healthy relationships but particularly in intimate relationships, as they allow you to be deeply intimate with your partner without losing sight of who you are.

Developing healthy boundaries

Boundaries are a strange concept to many people, perhaps because they are so inherent that we rarely acknowledge them – until someone crosses one! So why not just live with the boundaries we have? Because, unfortunately, they are not always conducive to healthy, happy relationships. As you read through the descriptions below, take time to reflect on whether your own boundaries are healthy and intact, non-existent, partially existent or fluctuating.

Because the idea of boundaries can sometimes be quite challenging at first (but also a revelation), I suggest reading through all of them, and writing notes and reflections on each type of boundary as you go along. It might be easier to do with a partner (or, if necessary, a counsellor or True Happiness group – see www.discovertruehappiness.com). For each boundary, reflect on how healthy yours currently are. Then reflect on the past: at what times have your, for example, physical boundaries, been infringed. Write down those incidents. When have you infringed other people's boundaries – write those down. If you feel upset as you do this, take time to gently process what you are feeling using the tools in Pillar Two (or with the help of a therapist). The ultimate purpose in doing this work is for you to live with healthy flexible boundaries. (Flexible boundaries simply means that you are able to adapt your boundaries to the situation you are in.) It's an essential task for true happiness.

There are four main boundaries – emotional, physical, intellectual and spiritual.

Emotional boundaries

Emotional boundaries refer to how you relate to others at the level of emotion. A person with healthy emotional boundaries (i.e. an emotionally mature adult):

- Takes full responsibility for their own emotions and for containing and expressing those emotions appropriately and respectively

- Does not take responsibility for another person's feelings, but takes them into consideration

- Is able to communicate their feelings to others in ways that own the feelings they have; for example, rather than using a statement starting, 'You . . . ' they use the words, 'I feel . . . '

- Are able to discriminate between their own feelings and those belonging to others

- Knows they have a right to any feeling that they are having, but not the right to use that feeling destructively against themselves or others

- Doesn't attempt to control or deny other people's feelings

- Determines the range of comments that they will accept from another person

- Will not infringe/disrespect another person's emotional boundaries (see below)

- Will set limits around anyone who infringes/disrespects their emotional boundaries (see below)

Infringement/disrespect of emotional boundaries

The most common ways in which emotional boundaries are infringed/disrespected include using feelings to manipulate another person (by using guilt or anger to try to control someone); diverting someone's attention when their feelings come up (for example, by switching subjects); minimising someone's feelings ('It's not that bad'); controlling another person's feelings ('Oh, just shut up'); discounting someone's feelings ('You are not really angry'); ignoring someone else's feelings (pretending you aren't aware of their feelings/emotional state); blaming your emotions on another person ('You make me feel mad') and so on.

Physical boundaries

Physical boundaries refer not only to parts of the physical body but also to your physical possessions. A person with healthy physical boundaries (i.e. an emotionally mature adult):

- Is able to know and communicate how physically close they want others to be with them

- Is able to know and communicate to others how they do or do not want to be touched

- Has the awareness to know when their physical boundaries are or have been infringed, and is able to take action in order to address this, usually in the form of a simple, respectful request

- Is able to communicate their sexual and non-sexual touch needs and desires to their partner and put limits in place if these are not respected

- Knows that no one has the right to touch them or be sexual with them without permission

- Will not infringe/disrespect another person's physical boundaries (see below)

- Will set limits around anyone who infringes/disrespects their physical boundaries (see below)

Infringement/disrespect of physical boundaries

Most of us are aware of the most serious infringements, for example committing sexual abuse and inflicting physical violence. However, there are many more subtle ways of violating physical boundaries, for example inappropriate sexual and non-sexual touch, invading someone's personal space without permission, unwanted tickling, listening to another person's conversations; not allowing others to have their personal space or privacy; taking someone's possessions without permission and so on.

Intellectual boundaries

Intellectual boundaries refer to your world view and perspective. This includes what you value, think, believe, want and need. A person with healthy intellectual boundaries (i.e. an emotionally mature adult):

- Takes responsibility for their own thoughts

- Values their own thoughts and opinions, but is open to those of others

- Will not sacrifice their own goals, wants and needs for someone else's without talking about it and negotiating a balance

- Will not infringe/disrespect another person's intellectual boundaries (see below)

- Will set limits around anyone who infringes/disrespects their intellectual boundaries (see below)

Infringement/disrespect of intellectual boundaries

The most common ways in which intellectual boundaries are infringed/disrespected include denying someone's perspective ('You are wrong'); patronising a person; interrupting someone while they are speaking; not listening to what the other person is saying; assuming that someone should see things the same way as you do; ignoring what someone has shared; ridiculing or berating someone; assuming you know what another person is thinking; saying, 'I know what is best for you'; saying, 'Lets not talk about that'.

Spiritual boundaries

Spiritual boundaries refer to your relationship with a transcendent higher power. They include your religion, spiritual beliefs and practices. A person with healthy spiritual boundaries (i.e. an emotionally mature adult):

- Knows and affirms their own spiritual nature and way of practising spirituality

- Will not infringe/disrespect another person's spiritual boundaries (see below)

- Will set limits around anyone who infringes/disrespects their spiritual boundaries (see below)

Infringement/disrespect of spiritual boundaries

The most common ways in which spiritual boundaries are infringed/disrespected include playing God ('You will do what I say'); portraying a condemning or judgemental picture of God ('You will burn in hell for that'); denying someone's right to different spiritual beliefs; denying someone's perspective ('You are wrong'); saying someone else's beliefs about the nature of reality are wrong; making out that you speak for God, questioning another person's faith or spiritual beliefs.

Tips for creating healthy boundaries

Boundaries work is vital to creating a positive, healthy relationship, but it is also highly sensitive. You can, however, make great inroads in developing healthy boundaries by doing the following:

- Increase your body awareness and emotional literacy (Pillar Two).

- Reflect back on your family and take an objective and honest look at the boundaries of each family member. What have you learnt? How have the early years impacted on your boundaries?

- Spend a day observing people's emotional boundaries, then the next day observing physical boundaries, then intellectual and then spiritual boundaries. Record your observations and discoveries in a notebook or journal.

- Read through the features of someone with healthy boundaries and start implementing them in your life.

- Practise communicating your needs and wants.

- Assume complete responsibility for your own thoughts, feelings and actions.

- Write down a list of all the fears you have about communicating your truth and setting boundaries.

- Create a list of your personal rights, making sure you cover each boundary type. For example, 'I have a right to say how and if I want to be touched.' Keep the list to hand so that you can remind yourself of your rights.

- If you struggle to speak your truth, try following the advice on assertiveness (see the box on page 260).

- Read some of the recommended books in the Resources (see page 291).

Boundaries work can be difficult for some people so you may also want to consider attending a workshop that teaches boundary skills (see Resources, page 288) or working with a counsellor or couples therapist to learn about boundaries.

Learn how to resolve conflicts

We all get into conflicts from time to time – it's inevitable. But the real challenge is knowing how to deal with them in a way that is life-affirming and that builds intimacy. If you haven't done so already, I encourage you to read the section on honest self-expression in Pillar Two (page 56), as this is at the heart of healthy conflict resolution.

The exercise below is an one that I share with people who want a safe, proven way to resolve conflict in a way that increases intimacy. It requires the input of both people concerned, however, so you will need the other person to agree to use it. Read through it a couple of times together, then try it next time you are in conflict.

EXERCISE: The respectful communication process

Awareness

- Become aware that you are stressed, tense or upset with your partner.

- Say something to them along the lines of, 'I need to share something important with you – is now a good time?'

- If it is, move on to the next step. If it isn't, agree exactly when would be a good time. As a general rule though, it is best to do this exercise after having processed the emotions you are feeling (see Pillars One and Two), especially if they are strong. This will increase the likelihood of this process working.

Active listening

- Sit down opposite each other.

- The person who has asked to do this exercise should take a few deep breaths and then start talking, while the other person listens.

- The person who is listening is going to use active listening. This, as its name suggests, means actively listening to the other person without interruption. The goal of the listener is to understand what is going on for the other person, by listening to them and trying to see things from their perspective.

- The person who is speaking needs to explain what is going on for them. One very effective and relatively non-threatening way to communicate is to use 'I' statements to communicate your feelings. Stay clear of character assassinations. For example, Mary saying to John: 'You have absolutely no respect for all the hard work I do around the house; you treat me like a slave; you are arrogant and selfish,' would become: 'I feel unappreciated at the moment. I'm really tired and exhausted with doing all the housework myself. If you could help me for just twenty minutes, twice a week, that would make me feel so much happier. It would demonstrate to me that you really care about me.'

- Once the message has been communicated, the listener needs to feed back the message in a way that demonstrates that they have genuinely understood the other person. At this stage, they don't have to agree with what has been said; they are just validating and acknowledging it.

- The listener then asks whether he or she has correctly understood everything. The first person either confirms that they have or communicates those areas that have been left out. The listener once again provides feedback.

- Now you reverse roles, and the other person shares their feelings.

Action

Once you have both communicated your feelings to each other, if it has been done effectively and genuinely, you should notice a shift in the energy between you. The focus is now on what specific action, if any, needs to be taken. Using the example of Mary and John above, they agreed that:

- John will help with the housework for twenty minutes every Saturday morning and Wednesday evening.

- When John gets home from work, rather than watching TV he will spend fifteen minutes with Mary, so they can talk about their respective days.

Appreciation

Once you've agreed on a plan of action, it's time to reconnect to each other. This could be anything from hugging, going for a walk, to kissing or making love – whatever works for you.

When arguments cross the threshold

From time to time, an argument may get out of hand. By this I mean that one of you feels emotionally overwhelmed, it is verbally abusive or potentially physically abusive. If any of these is the case, 'time out' can be called. This is a clear signal that this has gone too far and you can't cope.

On calling 'time out', all exchanges and communication must stop instantly. The person who called 'time out' must leave the room, but affirm that they are not leaving or threatening the relationship. Each person then must calm themself down, using tools that work for them. (See Anger, in Pillar Six, page 188.)

Once the person who called time out feels calm enough, they should return to the room with the other person and ask if they are ready to talk. If so, they should use the Respectful Communication Process (page 257).

LEARN HOW TO BE ASSERTIVE

Using the energy of anger in a way that allows you to communicate respectfully, clearly and maturely can have a very positive impact on your self-confidence and relationships. Let's face it, when we get angry with someone, say by shouting at them, we rarely get the result we want or, if we do, it doesn't usually feel 'clean' and healthy. Learning how to be assertive provides you with a great alternative, however, allowing you to communicate in a constructive, rather than destructive way.

Assertiveness is a give-and-take process. It involves:

- Presenting yourself authentically and being genuine and real

- Honouring and affirming your own truth, speaking your truth and receiving another person's truth

- Clearly, precisely and directly asking for what you want and need, then letting go of the need to control the outcome

- Saying no when you mean no, and saying yes when you mean yes

- Letting people know when they have hurt or offended you, and communicating that in a way that is respectful

- Being accountable for what you say and how you behave

Here are some suggestions to help you increase your assertiveness skills.

Take a risk and speak your truth   This can be difficult, but incredibly liberating once done. The key is to be clear about what your thoughts, feelings, needs and wants are and then to express them, with respect and without needing to control the outcome, despite the fear you might be feeling. Once spoken, try to listen to what is being said from the perspective of the person who is speaking to you. Stay connected to your own truth and respond once more. See honest self-expression (Pillar Two, page 56).

Try role play   With a trusted friend or even a practitioner, recreate a typical scenario that would lead to you becoming angry. Practise different ways of asserting yourself. Remember to breathe deeply. Tell your friend what it is you want. Practise changing your voice, your posture and your body language. Work out between you what works and rehearse it until it becomes your new way of relating.

Other tips for managing conflict

While being assertive and speaking your truth is an important part of creating healthy relationships, it needs to be balanced with listening and hearing the other person. Achieving this balance can be very challenging, but it comes with practice. Here are some additional suggestions for managing conflict.

- When you sense that conflict is about to happen or is happening immediately try and step into the shoes of the other person, and see things from their point of view. (See the section on empathy, page 237.)

- Focus on your breathing – breathe deeply and slowly – and listen to what the other person has to say.

- Drop the need to be right. Do you want to be right or in a relationship?

- Avoid the tendency to slip into defensive mode if that is what you usually do. Just focus on breathing and listening.

Contribute to the happiness and well-being of others

Dr Albert Schweitzer, doctor and Nobel Peace Prize winner once remarked, 'The only ones among you who will be really happy are those who have sought and found how to serve.' Research from a variety of sources is starting to confirm that his words are true. [111, 112, 113]

One of the most powerful ways to experience happiness and love is to be loving and caring towards others. This love and care can extend not just to our friends, partners and family but also to people we meet throughout our day. It might also involve volunteering our time and skills to causes greater than ourselves, such as a charity, club, society or community project. However, if we're totally honest, many of us give to get, though we're not necessarily fully aware of our motives. The key to discovering true happiness is to simply give to give, but to do so with awareness and in a way that is balanced. These two caveats are important. If we give without taking care of own health, well-being and responsibilities (such as our family), and/or if we are giving out of some unconscious need to belong or receive love and attention, then the giving is not healthy giving. It's unsustainable, it's imbalanced and it won't contribute to our happiness and well-being. It's inevitably going to lead to stress and possibly burn out, compassion fatigue and even illness. That's why awareness and balance are so important.

So why give?

Well, over and above the benefits to society, serving others (and our community) and giving is strongly associated with happiness, well-being and positive health. The American philosopher Ralph Waldo Emerson, in his famous essay on the topic of compensation, wrote, 'It is one of the most beautiful compensations of this life that no man can sincerely try to help another without helping himself'. Put another way, giving is receiving.

For me the 'giving is receiving' realisation has been a revelation, which is why I'm encouraging you to explore it. I invite many of my patients to try this and the vast majority report a very positive effect when they do so. Next time you perceive a 'lack' of something, whether it is love and attention from your partner, contact from a friend or lack of abundance, turn the situation around by asking yourself the following.

- What can I do to give love and attention to my partner? Now take action.

- Give your friend a call and tell them how much you value keeping in contact.

- Support someone else in creating abundance by whatever means are appropriate.

In a nutshell, anytime you think something is missing, and when appropriate (it isn't always), take actions to give that 'missing something' to someone else. Do this for one week and notice how it changes your perspective. It's a very powerful and enlightening experience and I really encourage you to discover its benefits for yourself.

And if you want some proof of the benefit of helping others, here's some fascinating research into the benefits of volunteering. A survey of 4,582 American adults found that 41 per cent of them had volunteered within the previous year.[114] Of those volunteers:

- 73 per cent agreed that 'volunteering lowers my stress levels'

- 89 per cent agreed that 'volunteering has improved my sense of well-being'

- 29 per cent who suffered from a chronic condition agreed that 'volunteering has helped me manage a chronic illness'

- 92 per cent agreed that volunteering enriches their sense of purpose in life

- 42 per cent said they have a 'very good' sense of meaning in their lives compared to 28 per cent of non-volunteers

Volunteering clearly provides many benefits to the recipients and to the volunteers. Here are some suggestions to support you in contributing to the well-being of others:

- Sign up with one of the many available online volunteering websites and commit to doing some regular voluntary work. Alternatively, find a local project that you can contribute a couple of hours per week/month to.

- Consider setting up a regular donation to a charity of your choice. While the benefit is less than if you were actively engaging with people within a volunteer setting, it can and does boost your happiness.[115]

- Over the next week do a couple of random acts of kindness – anything from offering to clean your neighbour's car, to buying someone a gift, volunteering or leaving a loving message for your partner. Look out also for opportunities to be kind spontaneously and in the moment. Like all skills, it takes practice and some creativity, but the results will be worth it. One of the knock-on benefits is the fact that kindness breeds kindness. If you are kind to others they are more likely to be kind to others too.[116]

PILLAR EIGHT: Summary

- One of our deepest needs is to feel connected to others and to have close, positive, healthy relationships.

- A healthy, positive relationship is any relationship between two people that is life-affirming and based on openness, honesty and mutual respect.

- To create a healthy, nourishing relationship, you need to learn the skills that will enable you to grow up.

- Empathy involves being fully present to another person with our whole being, while allowing ourself to fall into harmony and resonance with them.

- A significant barrier to intimacy is the presence of co- or counter-dependent behaviours, both of which have their origins in early childhood trauma.

- A boundary is an invisible fence or space that we put in place in order to protect ourselves and in order to maintain an authentic sense of self without offending others.

- Contributing to the well-being of others liberates true happiness from within.

A Final Word on True Happiness

Congratulations on getting to the end of this book! It takes considerable courage and commitment to do the work of waking up and growing up, so, even if you have implemented just a fraction of the suggestions in these pages, you should be proud of your accomplishments.

The deep sense of inner well-being, peace and vitality of true happiness is the gift that awaits you as you awaken to and embody your true self. True happiness is the reward you reap for switching from a way of being and living that is rooted in fear, guilt, limitation and conditioning, to one that is based on acceptance, awareness, love and contribution. By progressively learning how to accept all of your selves; by transforming the quality of your relationships, to your thoughts, emotions, to yourself and others; by taking action to address any underlying imbalances and barriers to emotional health and true happiness; and living life in alignment with your gifts, values and strengths in the service of the greater good, you can experience a truly fulfilling and meaningful life.

But all this takes work, patience and persistence! The key is committed daily action – doing something every day to wake up and grow up. And when you forget to do this (we are, after all, perfectly imperfect humans) be easy on yourself – just refocus and recommit to your happiness. With time, notice how much more effortless your life is becoming, and how happiness and the experience of well-being arise within you for no reason. This is the gift that awaits you.

At another level, the work of waking up and growing up is essential because humanity is heading towards a potential catastrophe if there isn't a significant shift in our attitudes, beliefs and the way we live our lives. Over-consumption and depletion of the earth's resources, global warming, the population explosion, rapidly approaching peak oil (the time at which global oil supplies reach a peak), the mass extinction of plant and animal species, nuclear threats and increasing poverty are bringing us to a critical juncture in time; one at which we must decide – individually and collectively – to stop acting like adolescents and start acting as mature adults who are responsible for our planet and for future generations.

We need a future that is sustainable. To make that happen we need people who are willing to give their gifts, talents, energy and time to a greater cause than just themselves. We need groups of like-minded, like-hearted people who are willing to co-operate and contribute to causes greater than themselves. Immature, 'asleep' adults can't do this because their focus is mainly on what they can get and take from the world. The focus and hallmark of a mature, awake adult, in contrast, is what they can give to and share with the world.

This is the crisis and the invitation of our time. Do we remain as emotional adolescents and endure the inevitable pain and suffering that comes with it? Or do we make a commitment to waking up, growing up and becoming emotionally mature adults who bring greater joy and harmony into the world?

It has been a pleasure to share my guide to true happiness with you.

Dr Mark Atkinson

**For more information on my course in True Happiness,
and how to set up a study group, plus much more,
visit www.discovertruehappiness.com**

Appendix
The 14-Day Happiness Test

So what is your real level of happiness? Here is one way to find out. Over the next fourteen days:

1. **Identify your emotional control strategies** (the different ways you sedate, control and avoid what you are feeling) and stop using them. Pillar Two (page 41) will show you how to do this. For most people this means giving up sugar, caffeine, alcohol, nicotine and using food to change the way you feel. It also means stopping judging others and yourself, refraining from gossiping, reducing your level of busyness and reducing the amount of TV you watch. Some of these, such as reducing sugar and caffeine intake for example, might need to be done slowly – say over a week or so.

2. **Start facing reality.** Do a life review – what part of your life are you not facing up to? Health? Relationships? Finances? Career? What are you avoiding? Take an honest look at the different areas of your life and start taking action to bring them into balance.

3. **Start breathing more deeply** (shallow breathing reduces emotional intensity) and throughout the day bring your awareness more fully into your body. Your emotions are located in your body – most people's awareness is limited to their head. See page 47.

Within 14 days of doing this, and usually earlier, you will discover for yourself the truth of how you are feeling. If strong uncomfortable emotions come up, as they often do, I recommend you use one or more of the tools that I outline in Pillars One and Two. These will help you work through what you are experiencing. (If you feel overwhelmed at anytime, I suggest you seek the help of a health professional.) A truly happy person will be at peace with whatever they are experiencing and will be aware of and feeling an undercurrent of gratefulness, joy and well-being most of the time in most situations.

Finally, if you know at the deepest level you aren't happy, but you are trying to convince yourself and others you are happy, you don't need to take the test – you simply need to admit it to yourself, at least one other person and start taking the actions outlined in this book.

References

1. Giltay, Erik J., Geleijnse, Johanna M., Zitman, Frans G., Hoekstra, Tiny, Schouten, Evert G., 'Dispositional optimism and all-cause and cardiovascular mortality in a prospective cohort of elderly Dutch men and women', *Archives of General Psychiatry*, Vol. 61 (2004), pp. 1126-35.
2. Fredrickson, B. L., 'The value of positive emotions', *American Scientist*, 91, (2003), pp. 330–35.
3. Gallup poll for *The Happiness Formula*, BBC 2 Series, Wednesday, 3 May 2006.
4. 'The World Health Report 2001: Mental Health: New Understanding, New Hope'; this can be downloaded from http://www.who.int/whr/2001/en/index.html.
5. Chatterji S., et al., 'Depression, chronic diseases, and decrements in health: Results from the World Health Surveys', *Lancet*, Vol. 370, Issue 9590 (2007), pp. 851–8.
6. Weinhold, Barry K. and Janae B., *The Flight from Intimacy*, New World Library (2008).
7. Griffin, Joe and Tyrrell, Ivan, *Human Givens: A New Approach to Emotional Well-Being and Clear Thinking*, Human Givens Publishing (2004).
8. Teasdale, John D., et al., 'Prevention of relapse/recurrence in major depression by mindfulness-based cognitive therapy', *Journal of Consulting and Clinical Psychology*, Vol. 68 (2000), No. 4, pp. 615–23.
9. Walsh Roger, 'Meditation practice and research', *Journal of Humanistic Psychology*, Vol. 23 (1983), No. 1, pp. 18–50.
10. Marcks, B. A., and Woods, D. W., 'A comparison of thought expression to an acceptance-based technique in the management of personal intrusive thoughts: A controlled evaluation', *Behaviour Research and Therapy*, Vol. 43 (2005), pp. 433–45.
11. Katie Byron, *Loving What Is*, Rider & Co (2002).
12. Griffin, J., Tyrrell, I., *Human Givens: A New Approach to Emotional Well-Being and Clear Thinking*, HG Publishing (2004).
13. Kashdan, Todd, et al., 'Experiential avoidance as a generalized psychological vulnerability: Comparisons with coping and emotion regulation strategies', *Behaviour Research and Therapy*, Vol. 44, Issue 9 (2006), pp. 1301–20.
14. Hayes, et al., *Acceptance and Commitment Therapy*, Guilford Press, 1st edition (2004).
15. Griffin J., Tyrell I., *Dreaming Reality: How Dreaming Keeps Us Sane, or Can Drive Us Mad*, HG Publishing, new edition (2006).
16. Sheldon K. M., and Elliot, A. J., 'Goal striving, need satisfaction and longitudinal well-being: The self-concordance model', *Journal of Personality and Social Psychology*, Vol. 76 (2004), pp. 546–7.
17. 'Research evidence of the effectiveness of self-care support' (work in progress 2005

to 2007), Department of Health; this report can be downloaded from www.dh.gov.uk.

18. Griffin, J. and Tyrrell, I., *Human Givens: A New Approach to Emotional Well-Being and Clear Thinking*, Human Givens Publishing (2004).

19. Brunstein, J. C., 'Personal goals and subjective well-being: A longitudinal study', *Journal of Personality and Social Psychology*, Vol. 65 (1997), pp. 1061–70.

20. Geary, A., *The Food and Mood Handbook*. Thorsons, illustrated edition (2001).

21. Holford, P., *Optimum Nutrition for the Mind*, Piatkus Books, new edition (2003).

22. 'The EWG shopper's guide to pesticides' report can be downloaded from http://www.foodnews.org/EWG-shoppers-guide-download-final.pdf.

23. Benton, B., 'The impact of the supply of glucose to the brain on mood and memory', *Nutrition Reviews*, Vol. 59(1 Pt 2) (2001), pp. S20–21.

24. Sofi, F., Cesari F., Abbate R., Gensini G. F., Casini A., 'Adherence to Mediterranean diet and health status: Meta-analysis', *BMJ (Clinical research edn)*, (2008)337: a1344.

25. Watkins, B. A., and Seifert, M. F., 'Food Lipids and Bone Health', in R. E. McDonald and D. B. Min (eds), *Food Lipids and Health*, Marcel Dekker, Inc., (1996) p. 101.

26. The Mental Health Foundation, Feeding Minds report (p. 10), www.mentalhealth.org.uk.

27. Tiemeier, H., et al., 'Plasma fatty acid composition and depression are associated in the elderly: The Rotterdam Study', *American Journal of Clinical Nutrition*, Vol. 78, (July 2003), No. 1, 40–46.

28. Rudin, D., 'The major psychoses and neuroses as omega-3 essential fatty acid deficiency syndrome: Substrate pellagra', *Biological Psychiatry*, Vol. 16, Issue 9 (1981), pp. 837–5.

29. Canty, D., Zeisel, S., 'Lecithin and choline in human health and disease', *Nutrition Reviews*, Vol. 52, Issue 10 (1994), pp. 327–39.

30. Haynes, A., *The Food Intolerance Bible*, Harper Thorsons (2005).

31. Meyer, K., et al., 'Carbohydrates, dietary fibre, and incident type 2 diabetes in older women', *American Journal of Clinical Nutrition*, Vol. 71, Issue 4 (April 2000), pp. 921–30.

32. Larsson, S., et al., 'Consumption of sugar and sugar-sweetened foods and the risk of pancreatic cancer in a prospective study', *American Journal of Clinical Nutrition*, Vol. 84, Issue 5 (November 2006), 11711–6.

33. Oomen, C., et al., 'Association between trans fatty acid intake and 10-year risk of coronary heart disease in the Zutphen Elderly Study: A prospective population-based study', *Lancet*, Vol. 357 (2001), pp. 746–51.

34. Walton, et al., 'Adverse reactions to aspartame: Double blind challenge in patients from a vulnerable population', *Journal of Biological Psychiatry*, Vol. 34(1–2) (1993), p. 13.

35. Tunnicliffe, J. M., Erdman, K. A., Reimer, R. A., Lun, V., Shearer, J., 'Consumption of dietary caffeine and coffee in physically active populations: Physiological interactions', *Applied Physiology, Nutrition & Metabolism*, Vol. 33, Issue 6 (December 2008), pp. 1301–10.

36. Food Standards Agency, 'National Diet & Nutrition Survey: Adults aged 19 to 64', Vol. 5 (2004).

37. 'Meat and dairy, where have the minerals gone?', *Food Magazine*, Vol. 72 (January/March 2006), p. 10.

38. Food Standards Agency, 'National Diet & Nutrition Survey: Adults aged 19 to 64', Vol. 5 (2004).

39. Benton, D., Roberts, G., 'Effect of vitamin and mineral supplementation on cognitive functioning', *Psychopharmacology* (Berl), Vol. 117, Issue (3) (1995), pp. 298–305.

40. Pearlstein, T., Steiner, M., 'Non-antidepressant treatment of premenstrual syndrome', *Journal of Clinical Psychiatry*, Vol. 61, Issue 12 (2000) pp. 22–7.

41. Toren, P., Eldar, S., Sela, B. A., et al., 'Zinc deficiency in attention-deficit hyperactivity disorder', *Biological Psychiatry* (1996), Vol. 40 (1996), pp. 1308–10.

42. Sugden, D., 'One carbon metabolism in psychiatric illness', *Nutrition Reviews*, Vol. 19 (2006), pp. 117–36.

43. Bottiglieri, T., 'Folate, vitamin B12, and neuropsychiatric disorders', *Nutrition Review* Vol. 54 (1996), pp 382–90.

44. Garg, H. K., et al., 'Zinc taste test in pregnant women and its correlation with serum zinc levels', *Indian Journal of Physiology & Pharmacology*, Vol. 37, Issue 4 (1993), pp. 318–22.

45. 'Medical aspects of exercise: Benefits and risks', summary of a report of the Royal College of Physicians, *Journal of the College of Physicians,* London, Vol. 25, Issue 3 (July 1991), pp. 193–6.

46. Babyak, M. A., Blumenthal, J. A., Herman, S., Khatri, P., Doraiswamy, P. M., Moore, K. A., Craighead, W. E., Baldewicz, T. T. and Krishnan, K. R., 'Exercise treatment for major depression: Maintenance of therapeutic benefit at 10 months', *Psychosomatic Medicine,* Vol. 62 (2003), pp. 633–8.

47. Lauderdale, et al., 'Respond to "How Much Do We Really Sleep?"', *American Journal of Epidemiology*, Vol. 164, Issue 1 (1 July 2006), pp. 19–20.

48. Institute of Medicine, www.ion.edu/sleep.

49. Johnson, E., 'Sleep in America 2000', National Sleep Foundation, www.sleepfoundation.org.

50. Benson, H., *The Relaxation Response*, Morrow (1976).

51. Jorde, R., et al., 'Effects of vitamin D supplementation on symptoms of depression in overweight and obese subjects: randomized double blind trial', *Journal of Internal Medicine*, Vol. 264, Issue 6 (December 2008), pp 599–609.

52. Llewellyn, D. J., Langa, K., Lang, I., 'Serum 25-Hydroxyvitamin D Concentration and Cognitive Impairment', *Journal of Geriatric Psychiatry and Neurology*, Vol. 22, Issue 3 (4 February 2009), pp. 188–95.

53. Baille-Hamilton, P., *Stop the 21st Century Killing You*, Vermilion (2005).

54. Coghill, R., *Electropollution: How to Protect Yourself Against It*, HarperCollins (1990).

55. Baille-Hamilton, P., *Stop the 21st Century Killing You*, Vermilion (2005).

56. Ibid.

57. Challem, J., *The Inflammation Syndrome: The Complete Nutritional Program to Prevent and Reverse Heart Disease, Arthritis, Diabetes, Allergies and Asthma*, John Wiley & Sons Inc. (2004).

58. Genthner, G. C., Friedman, H. L., Studley, C. F., 'Improvement in depression following reduction of upper cervical vertebral subluxation using orthospinology technique', *Journal of Vertebral Subluxation Research* (7 November 2005), pp. 1–4.

59. Coppen, A., 'The biochemistry of affective disorders', *British Journal of Psychiatry* (1967) 113:1237–64.

60. Poldinger, W., Calanchini, B., Shwarz, W., 'A functional-dimensional approach to depression: Serotonin deficiency as a target syndrome in a comparison of 5-hydroxytryptophan and fluvoxamine', *Psychopathology*, Vol. 24, *Psychopathology* (1991), pp. 53–81.

61. Harrer, G., Schmidt, U., Kuhn, U., Biller, A., 'Comparison of equivalence between

the St John's wort extract LoHyp-57 and fluoxetine', *Arzneimittelforschung*, Vol. 49 (1999), pp. 289–96.

62. Shiah, I. S., et al., 'GABA functions in mood disorders: An update and critical review', *Natural Life Sciences*, Vol. 63, Issue 15 (1998), pp. 1289–303.

63. Mason, R., '200mg of Zen; L-theanine boosts alpha waves, promotes alert relaxation', *Alternative & Complementary Therapies*, Vol. 7 (April 2001), pp. 91–5.

64. Habeck, M., 'New Insights into Alzheimer's Disease', *Drug Discovery Today*, Vol. 7, Issue 8 (2002), pp. 441–2.

65. Canty, D. J., et al., 'Lecithin and choline in human health and disease', *Nutrition Reviews*, Vol. 52, Issue 10 (1994), pp. 327–39.

66. Chung, S. Y., et al., 'Administration of phosphatidylcholine increases brain acetylcholine concentration and improves memory in mice with dementia', *Journal of Nutrition*, Vol. 125 (1995), pp. 1484–9.

67. Coppen, A., 'The biochemistry of affective disorders', *British Journal of Psychiatry*, Vol. 113 (1967), pp. 1237–64.

68. Beckman, H., et al., 'DL-phenylalanine versus imipramine: A double-blind controlled study', *Archiv für Psychiatrie und Nervenkrankheiten*, Vol. 227, Issue 1 (1979), pp. 49–58.

69. Benton, B., 'The impact of the supply of glucose to the brain on mood and memory', *Nutrition Review*, Vol. 59, No. 1, Pt 1 (2001), pp. S20–21.

70. Ebbesson, S. O., Risica, P. M., et al., 'Omega-3 fatty acids improve glucose tolerance and components of the metabolic syndrome in Alaskan Eskimos: The Alaska Siberia project', *International Journal* of *Circumpolar Health*, Vol, 64, Issue 4 (September 2005) pp. 396–408.

71. Anderson, R. A., Cheng, N., Bryden, N. A., et al., 'Elevated intakes of supplemental chromium improve glucose and insulin variables in individuals with type 2 diabetes', *Diabetes*, Vol. 46, Issue 11 (November 1997), pp. 1786–91.

72. Liu, J., et al., 'Memory loss in old rats is associated with brain mitochondrial decay and RNA/DNA oxidation: Partial reversal by feeding aceyl-l-carnitine and/or R-alpha- lipoic acid', *The Proceedings of the National Academy of Sciences*, Vol. 99, Issue 4 (19 February 2002), pp. 2356–61.

73. Hodgson, J. M., Watts, G. F., et al., 'Coenzyme Q10 improves blood pressure and glycaemic control: A controlled trial in subjects with type 2 diabetes', *European Journal of Clinical Nutrition*, Vol. 56, Issue 11 (November 2002), pp.1137–42.

74. Miller, J. W., 'Homocysteine and Alzheimer's disease', *Nutrition Review*, Vol 57, Issue 4 (April 1999), pp. 126–9.

75. Birmingham, C. L., et al. 'Controlled trial of zinc supplementation in anorexia nervosa', *International Journal of Eating Disorders*, Vol. 15, Issue 3 (April 1994), pp. 251–5.

76. Imada, Y., Yoshioka, S., Ueda, T., Katayama, S., Kuno, Y, Kawahara, R., 'Relationships between serum magnesium levels and clinical background factors in patients with mood disorders', *Psychiatry and Clinical Neurosciences*, Vol. 56 (2002), pp. 509–14.

77. Philpott, W., *Brain Allergies*, McGraw-Hill Contemporary, 2nd edition (2000).

78. Brown, R. P., Gerbarg, P. L., Ramazanov, Z., 'Rhodiola rosea: A phytomedicinal overview', *Herbalgram*, Vol. 56 (2002), pp. 40–52.

79. Wagner, H., Nörr, H., Winterhoff, H., 'Plant adaptogens', *Phytomed*, Vol. 1 (1994), pp 63–76.

80. Asano, K., Takahashi, T., Miyashita, M., et al., 'Effect of *Eleutherococcus senticosus* extract on human working capacity', *Planta Medica*, Vol. 37 (1986), pp. 175–7.

81. Duke, J., *Ginseng: A Concise Handbook,* Algonac, MI: Reference Publications (1989), pp. 36.

82. Vanderpump, M. P., Tunbridge, W. M., French, J. M., et al., 'The incidence of thyroid disorder in the community: A twenty-year follow-up of the Whickham survey', *Clinical Endocrinology*, Vol. 43 (1995), pp. 55–68.

83. Clark, C. D., Bassett, B., Burge, M. R., 'Effects of kelp supplementation on thyroid function in euthyroid subjects', *Endocrine Practice*, Vol. 9, Issue 5 (2003), pp. 363–9.

84. Loch, E. G., Selle, H., Boblitz, N., 'Treatment of premenstrual syndrome with a phytopharmaceutical formulation containing Vitex agnus castus', *Journal of Women's Health Gender Based Medicine*, Vol. 9, Issue 3 (2000), pp. 315–20.

85. Lieberman, S., 'A review of the effectiveness of *Cimicifuga racemosa* (black cohosh) for the symptoms of menopause', *Journal of Women's Health*, Vol. 7 (1998) pp. 525–9.

86. Han, K. K., Soares, J. M. Jr, Haidar, M. A., et al., 'Benefits of soy isoflavone therapeutic regimen on menopausal symptoms', *Obstetrics & Gynecology*, Vol. 99 (2002), pp. 389–94.

87. Di Silverio, F., Monti, S., Sciarra, A., et al., 'Effects of long-term treatment with Serenoa repens (Permixon®) on the concentrations and regional distribution of androgens and epidermal growth factor in benign prostatic hyperplasia', *Prostate*, Vol. 37 (1998), pp. 77–83.

88. Shippen, E., *The Testosterone Syndrome: The Critical Factor for Energy, Health and Sexuality: Reversing the Male Menopause*, M. Evans & Co. Inc. (2001).

89. Netter, A., Hartoma, R., Nahoul, K., 'Effect of zinc administration on plasma testosterone, dihydrotestosterone and sperm count', *Archives of Andrology*, Vol. 7, Issue 1 (August 1981), pp. 69–73.

90. Wilt, T. J., Ishani, A., Stark, G., et al., 'Saw palmetto extracts for treatment of benign prostatic hyperplasia', *JAMA*, Vol. 280 (1998), pp. 160–9.

91. Lipski, E., *Digestive Wellness*, McGraw-Hill Professional, 3rd edition (2004).

92. The World Health Report 2001, 'Mental Health: New Understanding, New Hope'; this can be downloaded from http://www.who.int/whr/2001/en/index.html.

93. Health and Safety Executive, www.hse.gov.uk/stress.

94. Wittchen, H. U., Hoyer, J., 'Generalized anxiety disorder: Nature and course', *Journal of Clinical Psychiatry*, Vol. 62, Supplement 11 (2001), pp. 15–19.

95. Ellsberg, M., 'Violence against women and the Millennium Development Goals: Facilitating women's access to support', *International Journal of Gynecology & Obstetrics*, Vol. 94, Issue 3 (2006), pp. 325–32.

96. Cawson, P., et al., 'Child maltreatment in the United Kingdom: A study of the prevalence of child abuse and neglect' (2000), London: NSPCC; this can be accessed at www.nspcc.org.uk.

97. Williams, L. M., 'Recall of childhood trauma: A prospective study of women's memories of child sexual abuse', *Journal of Consulting and Clinical Psychology*, Vol. 62 (1994), pp. 1167–76.

98. Heim, C., Nater, U. M., Maloney, E., Boneva, R., Jones, J. F., Reeves, W. C., 'Childhood trauma and risk for chronic fatigue syndrome: Association with neuroendocrine dysfunction', *Archives of General Psychiatry*, Vol 66, Issue 1 (2009), pp. 72–80.

99. Kubler-Ross, E. and Kessler, D., *On Grief and Grieving*, Simon & Schuster Ltd (2005).

100. Baumeister, R. F. and Leary, M. R., 'The need to belong: Desire for interpersonal attachments as a fundamental human motivation', *Psychological Bulletin*, Vol. 117 (1995), pp. 497–529.

101. Fowler, J., & Christakis, N. (2009), 'Dynamic spread of happiness in a large social network: Longitudinal analysis over 20 years in the Framingham Heart Study.' *British Medical Journal*, Vol. 338, Issue 7685, 1–13. 101.
102. Albrecht, K., *Social Intelligence: The New Science of Success*, Jossey-Bass (2006).
103. J. H., Medalie, et al., 'The importance of biopsychosocial factors in the development of duodenal ulcer in a cohort of middle-aged men,' *American Journal of Epidemiology*, Vol. 136 (1992), pp. 1280–87.
104. Giles, L., et al., 'Effect of social networks on 10-year survival in very old Australians: The Australian longitudinal study of aging', *Journal of Epidemiology and Community Health*, Vol. 59 (2005), pp. 574–9.
105. Orth-Gomer, K. and Johnson, J. V., 'Social network interaction and mortality: A six year follow-up study of a random sample of the Swedish population', *Journal of Chronic Diseases*, Vol. 40, Issue 10 (1987), pp. 949–57.
106. Fehr, B., *Friendship Processes*, Sage Publications, Inc. (1996).
107. Fredrickson, B., Cohn, M., Coffey, K. A., Pek, J. and Finkel, S. M., 'Open hearts build lives: positive emotions, induced through loving-kindness meditation, build consequential personal resources', *Journal of Personality and Social Psychology*, Vol. 95, Issue 5 (2008), pp. 1045–62.
108. Gottman, J. M., Coan, J., Carrere, S., Swanson, C., 'Predicting marital happiness and stability from newlywed interactions', *Journal of Marriage and the Family*, Vol. 60, Issue 2 (1998), pp. 5–22.
109. Weinhold, B. K. and J. B., *The Flight from Intimacy*, New World Library (2008).
110. Bowlby, J., *A Secure Base*, Routledge, 1st edition (1 September 2005).
111. Arnstein, P., Vidal, M., Well-Federman, C., Morgan, B., Caudill, M., 'From chronic pain patient to peer: Benefits and risks of volunteering', *Pain Management Nurses*, Vol. 3, Issue 3 (2002) pp. 94–103.
112. Bachner-Melman, R., Gritsenko, I., Nemanov, L., Zohar, A. H., Dina, C., and Ebstein, R. P., 'Dopaminergic polymorphisms associated with self-report measures of human altruism: A fresh phenotype for the dopamine D4 receptor', *Molecular Psychiatry*, Vol 10 (2005), pp. 333–5.
113. Dulin, P. and Hill, R., 'Relationships between altruistic activity and positive and negative affect among low-income older adult service providers', *Aging & Mental Health*, Vol. 7, Issue 4 (2003), pp. 294–9.
114. www.unitedhealthgroup.com/news/rel2010/UHC-VolunteerMatch-Survey-Fact-Sheet.pdf Gottman, J.
115. Dunn, E. W., Aknin, L.B., Norton, M. I.,. 'Spending money on others promotes Happiness', *Science*, Vol. 319, Issue 5870 (21 March 2008) pp. 1687–8.
116. Fowler, J., et al., 'Cooperative behavior cascades in human social networks.' *Proceedings of the National Academy of Sciences*, Vol. 107, Issue 10, March 9, 2010.

Resources

Workshops/training courses

The Academy of Human Potential
Website: www.humanpotential.uk.com
Telephone: 0845 0948612

Human potential coaches
Trained by myself, they can support and mentor you through your
   true happiness programme
Website: www.humanpotential.uk.com
Telephone: 0845 0948612

Health practitioners and organisations – UK

If you need help and advice in overcoming a health or emotional
challenge, I recommend that you contact one of the following organ-
isations:

My own private practice
Website: www.drmarkatkinson.com
Telephone: 0845 0948612

British Society of Integrated Medicine
For doctors who practise integrative medicine
Website: www.bsim.org.uk
Telephone: 01962 718000

British Society for Ecological Medicine
For doctors who practise allergy, environmental and nutritional medicine
Website: www.ecomed.org.uk
Telephone: 0207 100 7090

Complementary Medical Association
The world's largest membership organisation for complementary therapists
Website: www.the-cma.org.uk
Telephone: 0845 1298434

British Naturopathic Association
The professional body for naturopaths
Website: www.naturopaths.org.uk
Telephone: 0870 7456984

British Association of Nutritional Therapists
The professional body for nutritional therapists
Website: www.bant.org.uk
Telephone: 08706 061284

Human Givens Therapists
The professional register of Human Givens therapists
Website: www.hgi.org.uk/register/
Telephone: 01323 811662

Health practitioners – worldwide

Australasian Integrative Medical Association
Provides a list of general practitioners and/or specialists who are members of the association and who practise some form of integrative medicine
Website: www.aima.net.au
Telephone: (03) 86990582

New Zealand Natural Medicine Association
Provides a list of health professionals dedicated to the promotion of
integrative healthcare
Website: www.nznma.com
Telephone: (09) 4432066

South African Society of Integrative Medicine
Provides a list of registered health practitioners who practise, or
have an interest in, integrative medicine
Website: www.integrativemedicine.co.za
Telephone: (021) 8851010

American Association of Integrative Medicine
Provides a list of health professionals dedicated to the promotion of
integrative healthcare
Website: www.aaimedicine.com
Telephone: (877) 7183053

American Holistic Medical Association
Provides a list of health professionals dedicated to the promotion of
holistic healthcare
Website: www.holisticmedicine.org
Telephone: (216) 2926644

Supplement companies/suppliers – UK

Higher Nature
One of the UK's leading supplement companies
Website: www.highernature.co.uk
Telephone: 0800 4584747

Nutricentre
A mail order and retail company selling high-quality supplements
(also foods, books and CDs)
Website: www.nutricentre.com
Telephone: 0845 602 6744

Revital

A mail order and retail company selling high-quality supplements (also foods, books and CDs)

Website: www.revital.com

Telephone: 0800 252875

Nutrilink

A supplier of nutritional supplements to practitioners

Website: www.nutri-linkltd.co.uk

Telephone: 0845 0760402

Supplement companies – worldwide

Higher Nature

Delivers products worldwide

Website: www.highernature.co.uk.

Blackmores (Australia)

Website: www.blackmores.com.au

Telephone: (02) 99105000

Bioharmony (South Africa)

Website: www.bioharmony.co.za

Telephone: (0860) 888339

Nature's Plus (USA)

Website: www.naturesplus.com

Telephone: (800) 6459500

Allergy Research Group (USA)

Website: www.allergyresearchgroup.com

Telephone: (800) 5459960

Diagnostic testing – UK

Genova Diagnostics Europe

Website: www.gdx.uk.net

Telephone: 020 8336 7750

Candida/parasite testing
Website: www.candidatest.co.uk
Telephone: 0844 330 1909

Diagnostic testing – worldwide

Nutritional Laboratory Services (Australia)
Website: www.nlabs.com.au
Telephone: (1300) 734413

Online Natural Pharmacy (New Zealand)
Website: www.healthyonline.co.nz
Telephone: (0800) 432 584

Molecular Diagnostic Services (South Africa)
Website: www.mdsafrica.net
Telephone: (31) 5224762

Genova Diagnostics (USA)
Website: www.genovadiagnostics.com
Telephone: (800) 5224762

Recommended Websites, Supplements and Products

All of the supplements mentioned in this section can be purchased from:

- Higher Nature (www.highernature.co.uk/0800 4584747)

- Nutrilink (www.nutri-linkltd.co.uk/0870 4054002)

- Nutricentre (www.nutricentre.com/0845 6026744)

- Revital (www.revital.com/0800 252875)

Pillar One: Get out of your head

- If you want to go even deeper with the 'getting out of your head' work, I recommend Leo Hawkins's approach to present-moment awareness. Leo Hawkins www.breakoutofyourmind.com

- Mindfulness CDs: *Guided Meditations: For Calmness, Awareness and Love* by Bodhipaska (from Amazon); *Guided Mindfulness Meditation* by Jon Kabat-Zinn (from Amazon)

- The Work: www.thework.com (website of Byron Katie)

- I highly recommend Richard Miller's version of yoga nidra, a form of meditation practice that trains you to welcome reality as it is. His website is www.irest.us

- Website of Arjuna Ardagh: www.livingessence.com. Arjuna is an inspirational teacher who has written extensively about people 'waking up' and experiencing 'translucence' – a deeper purpose and presence and a sense of joy.

Pillar Two: Become a master of your emotions

- Human Givens Institute website: www.hgi.org.uk (provides details of qualified Human Givens therapists)

- EmoTrance www.emotrance.com (provides more information on EmoTrance and a list of EmoTrance practitioners)

- Breathwork: www.drmarkatkinson.com; www.rebirthingbreathwork.co.uk (for breathwork courses and workshops)

- Emotional Clearing is a very effective way to work with emotion. Developed by John Ruskan, it complements my approach well: www.emclear.com

Pillar Three: Live a fulfilling and meaningful life

- My Total Well-being Club and workshops www.drmarkatkinson.com

- The Hoffman Process, www.hoffmaninstitute.org. They offer an eight-day personal development workshop, which I have found – having done it myself – can deepen and accelerate the process of growing up and waking up.

- Anthony Robbins is the world's most famous personal development expert: www.tonyrobbins.com

- Gay and Kathleen Hendricks, www.hendricks.com. Gay Hendricks is a leading pioneer in conscious living and he and his wife Kathleen have written extensively about conscious loving and relationships – they're both truly inspirational.

Pillar Four: Meet your physical needs

Sleep

- Alpha-Stim SCS and Guided Imagery CD: www.mindbodyproducts.com

Relaxation

- Mindfulness classes: www.bangor.ac.uk/mindfulness

Healthy environment

- Natural cleaning products: Natural House (www.natural-house.co.uk) and 21st Century Health (www.21stcenturyhealth.co.uk)

- Personal care products: Neal's Yard Remedies (www.nealsyardremedies.com), The Green People Company (www.greenpeople.co.uk) and Goodness Direct (www.goodnessdirect.co.uk)

- Water filters: Santevia water system (www.healthyandessentialwater.com), wellness filter system (www.highernature.co.uk) or a reverse-osmosis system (www.freshlysqueezedwater.org.uk) will provide you with clean water, free from contaminants. If you use the latter system you should add minerals back in (see www.eletewater.co.uk).

- Full-spectrum lighting www.lifeliteuk.com

- The British Society of Mercury-free Dentists: www.mercuryfreedentistry.org.uk

Nutrition

- Help for eating disorders: www.eating-disorders.org.uk

- Metabolic typing: www.metabolictyping.com

- Mineral test kits: www.mineraltestkit.co.uk/

- Protein shakes: Higher Nature's High Fibre Vitality Shake or Energy Breakfast Shake or Hemp Protein Powder www.highernature.co.uk

Foundation supplement programme

- **Multivitamin–mineral:** Advanced Nutrition Complex (from Higher Nature) or Allergy Research MVM-Antioxidant from Nutrilink

- **Vitamin C:** Higher Nature's Calcium Ascorbate Powder or Allergy Research Ester-C from Nutrilink

- **Fish Oil:** Nordic Naturals Arctic Omega – Liquid (from Nutrilink), Barleans Omega Swirl (from www.healthyandessential.com) or Emulsified Fish Oil (from Higher Nature) or Organic Flaxseed Oil if vegetarian (from Higher Nature) or Organic Omega 3:6:9 Balance Oil (from Higher Nature)

- **Wholefood supplement:** Easy-3 (from Higher Nature)

Pillar Five: Identify and address physical imbalances

- All of the recommended tests in this section are from Genova Diagnostics www.gdx.uk.net

- Candida test is from www.candidatest.co.uk

Neurotransmitter imbalances

- **5-HTP:** Higher Nature's Serotone 5-HTP or Higher Nature's Positive Outlook (which also contains l-tyrosine), or Higher Nature's St John's Wort or Bioforce A.Vogel Hypericum (St John's Wort)

- **GABA:** Higher Nature's L-theanine or Higher Nature's Balance for Nerves (contains l-theanine, passion flower and lemon balm) or Zen from Nutrilink (contains GABA and l-theanine)

- **Acetylcholine:** Higher Nature's High PC Lecithin and/or Higher Nature's Advanced Brain Nutrients (includes choline, phosphatidyl serine and acetyl-l-carnitine); alternatively Allergy Research Phosphatidyl Choline from Nutrilink

- **Dopamine:** Higher Nature's Drive (contains tyrosine) or Higher Nature's Positive Outlook (contains 5-HTP and l-tyrosine); alternatively Allergy Research L-Tyrosine from Nutrilink or Solgar's L-Phenyalanine from Revital/NutriCentre

Nutritional imbalances
Dysglycemia

- Higher Nature's Chromium GTF or Higher Nature's Chromium polynicotinate or Allergy Research Sugar Balance Formula from Nutrilink (contains chromium, alpha lipoic acid and a proprietary blend of sugar-stabilising ingredients)

- Higher Nature's Alpha (contains alpha lipoic acid) or sugar balance formula (see above)

- Higher Nature's Coenzyme Q10 or Allergy Research Coenzyme Q10 from Nutrilink

- Higher Nature's Glutamine or Allergy Research L-Glutamine from Nutrilink

Others

- Homocysteine test: from Genova Diagnostics www.gdx.uk.net

- B-vitamin imbalance: Higher Nature's H-Factors (contains TMG, vitamin B_2, B_6, B_{12} and folic acid) or Allergy Research Homocysteine Metabolite Formula from Nutrilink

- Zinc: Higher Nature's Sublingual Zinc or Allergy Research Zinc Picolinate from Nutrilink or Metagenics Zinc Drink from Revital/NutriCentre

- Magnesium: Higher Nature's True Food Magnesium or Allergy Research Solution of Magnesium (liquid form) from Nutrilink

Allergies/intolerances

- Higher Nature's Glutamine or Allergy Research Perm A vite powder from Nutrilink (contains glutamine, slippery elm and N-acetyl-D-glucosamine); Higher Nature's Supergest or Biotics Intenzyme Forte from Nutrilink (these are both digestive enzymes); Higher Nature's ProbioIntensive or Allergy Research GI Flora from Nutrilink (both of these are probiotics); Higher Nature's Aloe Gold or Donsbach Aloe Vera Juice from Revital/NutriCentre

Hormone imbalances

- Adrenals: Higher Nature's Rhodiola and Ashwaghanda or Higher Nature's B-Vital (contains ginseng) or Allergy Research Dr Wilson's Dynamite Adrenal Powder from Nutrilink (contains a proprietary blend of ingredients to support the adrenals – you won't need to take a multivitamin while taking this product)

- Thyroid: Higher Nature's Thyroid Support Formula (contains tyrosine) or Higher Nature's Ocean Kelp or Allergy Research TG 100 Organic Glandulars from Nutrilink

- Information on Amour Thyroid: Thyroid UK www.thyroiduk.org

- Oestrogen/progesterone: Higher Nature's Dong Quai and Agnus Castus or Allergy Research DIM Vitex (contains agnus castus); Bioforce A.Vogel Black Cohosh Complex from Revital/NutriCentre or Allergy Research Women's Prime (contains black cohosh); Higher Nature's True Food Super Potency Soyagen (fermented soya); Higher Nature's Saw Palmetto and Pygeum Bark or Allergy Research Palmetto Complex II with Lycopene from Nutrilink

- Testosterone: Higher Nature's Sublingual Zinc *or* Allergy Research Zinc Picolinate from Nutrilink *or* Metagenics Zinc Drink from Revital/NutriCentre; Higher Nature Saw Palmetto and Pygeum Bark or Allergy Research Palmetto Complex II with Lycopene from Nutrilink

Dysbiosis

- Tests from Genova Diagnostics www.gdx.uk.net

- Higher Nature's Paraclens or Dulwich Health Oxytech (www.dulwichhealth.co.uk) or Allergy Research Tricycline from Nutrilink (contains berberine, artemisinin, citrus seed extract)

- Probiotics: Higher Nature's ProbioIntensive or Allergy Research GI Flora from Nutrilink

- Immune Support: Cordyceps, Maitake, Reishi, Shiitake and Trametes Complex (from Fruiting Bodies: www.fruiting-bodies.co.uk) or Biobran MGN-3 from Revital/NutriCentre

- Alkaline mineral salts – product name: Alkaclear (from Higher Nature) and milk thistle and artichoke (also from Higher Nature)

Pillar Six: Identify and address mental-health challenges

Psychological stress

- HeartMath Institute: www.heartmath.org

- Recommended music: Medical Resonance Therapy Music www.medicalresonancetherapymusic.com; Jacotte Chollet www.multidimensionalmusic.com; John Levine www.silenceofmusic.com; Steven Halpern www.innerpeacemusic.com

- Spring Forest Qi Gong: www.springforestqigong.com

- Bach flower remedies. www.nelsons.net/en-gb/

Depression

- Therapists: Human Givens therapists: www.hgi.org.uk; cognitive behavioural therapist: www.babcp.com; solution-focused brief therapy: www.brieftherapy.org.uk; and acceptance and commitment therapy: www.contextualpsychology.org

- Alpha-Stim and CDs: www.mindbodyproducts.com

- SAD lightboxes: www.sadbox.co.uk

- Depression Alliance: www.depressionalliance.org

- Self-help depression programmes: www.clinical-depression.co.uk and www.moodgym.anu.edu.au

Anxiety and panic disorder

- Online anxiety management course: www.moodgym.anu.edu.au

- Alpha-Stim SCS: www.mindbodyproducts.com

- Social Anxiety UK: http://www.social-anxiety.org.uk/

- Anxiety Care: www.anxietycare.org.uk

- MIND: www.mind.org.uk

- Rewind technique: www.rewindtechnique.com/

- Therapists: Human Givens therapist: www.hgi.org.uk; cognitive behavioural therapist: www.babcp.com; solution-focused brief therapy: www.brieftherapy.org.uk; and acceptance and commitment therapy: www.contextualpsychology.org

Addictions

- Alliance for Addiction Solutions www.allianceforaddictionsolutions.org

- Promis Addictive Tendencies Questionnaire: www.s-p-q.com

- Information on twelve-step support groups: www.12step.org

- Alcoholics Anonymous: www.alcoholics-anonymous.org.uk_

- Al-Anon (for partners of people with alcohol addiction) www.al-anonuk.org.uk

- For information on the SMART recovery programme visit: www.smartrecovery.org

- UK treatment centres: Bayberry Clinic (for professionals): www.bayberryclinic.org.uk; Prinsted www.prinsted.org, Life-Works: www.lifeworkscommunity.com; Linwood Group www.lynwodemanor.co.uk; Action on Addiction: www.actiononaddiction.org.uk.

- USA treatment centres: the Bridge to Recovery: www.thebridgetorecovery.com; the Ranch www.recoveryranch.com; the Meadows: www.themeadows.org; Pine Grove (sex addiction) www.pinegrovetreatment.com; and Caron www.caron.org.

- Other treatment centres: Montrose Place (South Africa) www.montroseplace.co.za/, Montrose Manor (South Africa) (eating disorders) www.montrosemanor.co.za/ Crossroads (Antigua); www.crossroadsantigua.org; Tabankulu (South Africa) www.tabankulu.co.za;

- Holistic Addictions Treatment Programme www.drmarkatkinson.com (see consultation section) NHS Smoke Free: www.smokefree.nhs.uk/

Trauma/PTSD

- Trauma therapies: the rewind technique www.hgi.org.uk/register/, EMDR www.emdrassociation.org.uk, trauma release process www.traumaprevention.com and somatic experiencing www.traumahealing.com

Grief

- **Grief Recovery Institute**: www.grief.net

Pillar Seven: Accept and love yourself

- Working with the selves – The True Happiness workshop www.discovertruehappiness.com

- Website of Hal and Sidra Stone: www.delos-inc.com

- Website of Dennis Genpo Merzel www.bigmind.org

Pillar Eight: Create healthy, positive relationships

- Co-dependency treatment: the Bridge to Recovery in Bowling Green, Kentucky, USA: www.thebridgetorecovery.com

- Recommended workshop providers: The Academy of Human Potential (www.humanpotential.uk.com), Onsite (www.onsiteworkshops.com), the Hoffman Process (www.hoffmaninstitute.co.uk), the Meadows (www.themeadows.org), Caron (www.caron.org) and Heart Stream Journeys (www.heartstreamjourneys.com)

- Workshops/consultations with Barry and Janae Weinhold: www.weinholds.org

- Emotionally focused therapy: www.eft.ca

- Co-dependents Anonymous (CODA): www.codependents.org

- Recovering Couples Anonymous www.recovering-couples.org

- Empathy training: www.compassionatecommunication.co.uk, www.cnvc.org/

- Relationship Counsellors: www.relate.org.uk

- 'The Healing Power of Loving-Kindness: A Guided Buddhist Meditation' (Book and CD) by Tulku Thondup (from Amazon).

Recommended Reading

Pillar One: Get out of your head

Meditation for Dummies, 2nd edition, John Wiley & Sons (2006)
Tolle Eckart, *Practising the Power of Now*, Mobius (2002)
Hawkins, Leo, *Break out of your mind*, Global Alchemy Publishing (2009)
Kabat-Zinn, Jon, *Full Catastrophe Living*, Piatkus Books (2001)
Byron, Katie, *Loving What Is*, Rider & Co (2002)
Ardagh, Arjuna, *The Translucent Revolution*, New World Library; First Printing, Highlighting edition (2005)
Miller, Richard, *Yoga Nidra*, Sounds True Inc; Har/Com edition (2005)

Pillar Two: Become a master of your emotions

Atkinson, Mark, *The Mind–Body Bible*, Piatkus Books (2007)
Simon, David, *Free to Love, Free to Heal*, Chopra Center Press (2010)
Brown, Michael, *The Presence Process: A Journey Into Present Moment Awareness*, Namaste Publishing; 2nd edition (2010)
Ruskan, John, *Emotional Clearing*, Rider & Co (1998)

Pillar Three: Live a fulfilling and meaningful life

Griffin, Joe and Tyrrell, Ivan, *Human Givens: A New Approach to Emotional Well-Being, Health and Clear Thinking*, Human Givens Publishing (2004)
Hendricks, Gay, *The Big Leap*, HarperOne (2009)

Pillar Four: Meet your physical needs

Atkinson, Mark, *The Mind–Body Bible,* Piatkus Books (2007)
Null, Gary, *Food–Mood–Body Connection*, 2nd edition, Seven Stories Press (2008)

Pillar Five: Identify and address physical imbalances

Atkinson, Mark, *The Mind–Body Bible,* Piatkus Books (2007)
Holford, Patrick, *Optimum Nutrition for the Mind*, Piatkus Books (September 2003)

Pillar Six: Identify and address any mental-health challenges

Psychological stress

Childre, Doc, *The Heartmath Solution*, 1st edition, HarperOne (2000)
Colbert MD, Don, *Stress Less*, Siloam Press (2005)

Anger

Carter, Les, *The Anger Trap: Free Yourself from the Frustrations that Sabotage Your Life*, Jossey Bass (2004)
Griffin, Joe and Tyrrell, Ivan, *Release from Anger*, Human Givens Publishing (2008)

Anxiety and panic disorders

Griffin, Joe and Tyrrell, Ivan, *How to Master Anxiety: All You Need to Know to Overcome Stress, Panic Attacks, Trauma, Phobias, Obsessions and More*, HG Publishing (2006)
Peurifoy, Reneau Z., *Anxiety Phobia and Panic: A Step-by-step Programme for Regaining Control of Your Life*, Piatkus Books (2006)

Depression

Baumel, Syd, *Dealing with Depression Naturally,* 2nd edition, McGraw-Hill Contemporary (2000)
Griffin, Joe and Tyrell, Ivan, *How to Lift Depression Fast*, HG Publishing (2004)

Addictions

Kasl, Charlotte D., *Women, Sex and Addiction: A Search for Love and Power*, Harper Perennial (1990)

Mellody, Pia, *Facing Love Addiction*, Harper San Francisco (2003)

Trauma/PTSD

Berceli, David, *The Revolutionary Trauma Release Process*, Namaste Publishing Inc (2008)

Levine, Peter, *Healing Trauma*, Sounds True (2005)

Grief

James, John and Friedman, Russell, *The Grief Recovery Handbook*, 20th anniversary edition, Collins (2009)

Kubler-Ross, Elizabeth and Kessler, David, *On Grief and Grieving*, Simon & Schuster Ltd (2005)

Pillar Seven: Accept and love yourself

Hendricks, Gay, *Learning to Love Yourself Workbook*, Prentice Hall & IBD (1993)

Luskin, Fred, *Forgive for Good*, reprint edition, Harper San Francisco (2003)

Stone, Hal, *Embracing Our Selves*, Nataraj Publishing; New edition (1989)

Merzel, Dennis Genpo, *Big Mind, Big Heart*, Gazelle Drake Publishing; Pap/Com edition (2007)

Pillar Eight: Create Positive, Healthy Relationships

Richo, David, *How to be an Adult in Relationships*, Shambhala Publications Inc; 1st edition (2002)

Rosenburg, Marshall, *Nonviolent Communication*, Puddle Dancer Press; 2nd Revised edition (2003)

Litvinoff, Sarah, *Relate Guide to Sex in Loving Relationships*, Vermilion (2001)

Weinhold, Janae B. and Barry K., *The Flight from Intimacy*, New World Library (2008)

Weinhold, Janae B. and Barry K., *Breaking Free of the Co-dependency Trap*, New World Library; 2nd Revised edition (2008)

Index

value-based goals 85–7
eye-movement desensitisation
 and reprocessing (EMDR) 205

fats and oils 100
fermented soya 99, 164, 165, 284
5-HTP 115, 141–2, 282, 283
Flight from Intimacy, The
 (Weinhold) 247
Florence (case study: seeking
 guidance) xx
fluctuating blood sugar
 (dysglycemia) 129–30, 147,
 158, 161, 164, 167, 194, 198,
 283; *see also* blood sugar
 addressing underlying causes of
 148
 dietary adjustments for 149
Food Standards Agency 106
forgiveness 219–20
four As of healthy relationships
 241–5
 acceptance 242–3
 affection 244–5
 appreciation 243–4
 attention 241–2
fourteen-day happiness test
 14–15, 267–8
Fredrickson, Prof. Barbara 2
Freeze Frame 186
friendship, power of 236
fulfilment and meaning, *see* Pillar
 Three

GABA 126, 127, 140, 142–3, 162,
 198
 dietary adjustments to boost
 143
 low, addressing underlying
 causes of 143
 low, questionnaire for 127
gateway 231
gaze xxiv
getting 'out of your head', *see*
 Pillar One
ginseng 159

Gloria (case study: disconnection)
 233–4
gratitude 62, 72–4
 exercises for 73–5
gratitude 62, 72–4
grief 181, 206–9, 287
 breathwork for 208
 communicating 208
 crying over 208
 process of 206–7
 processing, suggestions for
 207–8
 professional help for 209
 questionnaire for 181
 seminars for 208
 talking/feeling through 208
 tools and techniques for 208–9
 unresolved, signs and
 symptoms of 207
Griffin, Joe 52
growing up 5–7, 10

happiness:
 chain reaction to xx–xxi
 choosing 18–19
 ego and 6
 explained 3–4
 fourteen-day test for 14–15,
 267–8
 growing up to feel 5
 importance of 1–2
 maximising xviii–xix
 no appreciable improvement in
 3
 obstacles to 5
Hashimoto's disease 160
health-depleting foods
 alcohol 104–5
 caffeine 104
 intolerance 102
 refined carbohydrates 102
 sugar 103
 sweeteners 103–4
 trans fats 103
health-promoting foods 97–101
 amino acids 99–100

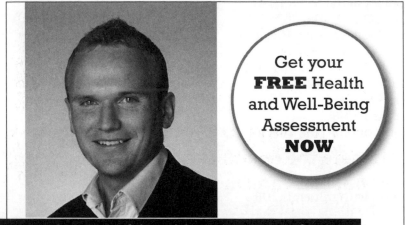

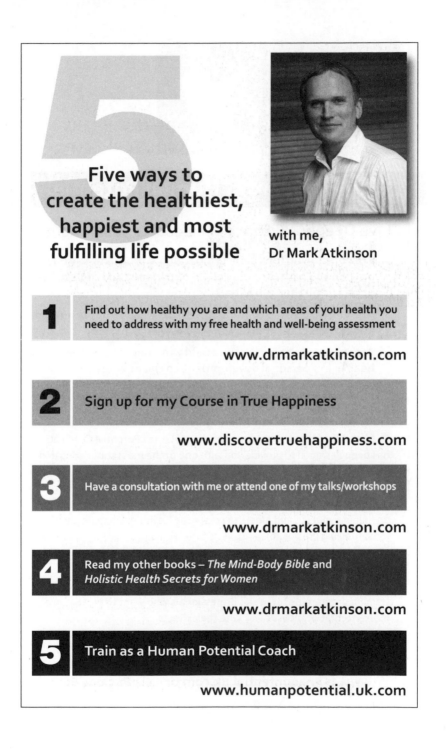

Five ways to create the healthiest, happiest and most fulfilling life possible

with me, Dr Mark Atkinson

1 Find out how healthy you are and which areas of your health you need to address with my free health and well-being assessment

www.drmarkatkinson.com

2 Sign up for my Course in True Happiness

www.discovertruehappiness.com

3 Have a consultation with me or attend one of my talks/workshops

www.drmarkatkinson.com

4 Read my other books – *The Mind-Body Bible* and *Holistic Health Secrets for Women*

www.drmarkatkinson.com

5 Train as a Human Potential Coach

www.humanpotential.uk.com

The Academy of **Human Potential**

Live Deeply – *Create a Life Equal to your Potential*

✓ Are you looking for a pioneering training programme that will provide you with the knowledge, experience and tools to help others fulfill their potential?

✓ Are you interested in holistic health, well-being, the mind-body connection and personal growth?

✓ Are you ready to enrich the quality of your life and take your health and personal development to the next level?

Human Potential Coach Training

Dr Mark Atkinson's training programme in Human Potential Coaching has been designed to provide you with one of the most stimulating and innovative coaching courses in the world. Training as a Human Potential Coach provides an unprecedented opportunity to enrich your life by having a deeply fulfilling and rewarding career which is focused on helping yourself and others to create the healthiest, happiest and most fulfilling life possible.

Integral Well-Being Therapy

Integral Well-Being Therapy is Dr Mark Atkinson's flagship professional training programme for health professionals who want to practise in a more integrative, holistic way with their clients.

For more information visit
www.humanpotential.uk.com or call **0845 094 8612**